# *The Mindful Path:*
## Combining Psychotherapy and Buddhist Practices

A Practical Guide for
Overcoming Anxiety, Depression, and Stress

Michael Jones, Ph.D.

Book Cover by Damonza.com

Book Design and Illustrations by Doriana Del Pilar

First edition 2023

ISBN 979-8-9882440-1-1

Library of Congress Control Number: 2023907918

# TABLE OF CONTENTS

# INTRODUCTION

People read a book for a variety of reasons. It may be simple curiosity or a random gift from a friend. However, I suspect you are reading this book because you are on a journey. Your journey is your desire to move toward a life that has more consistent happiness and well-being. This is the journey for most of us.

You may feel stressed at home or at work. You may suffer from a mental health problem like anxiety, depression, anger, or posttraumatic stress. Your situation may include coming to terms with difficult experiences you have had along your journey. You may think about trying therapy but are not yet sure. Or, you may have already tried therapy but felt like something was missing or it didn't help. You may have read spiritual books, but they left you unsure how to apply the ideas. If any of these things apply, this book is for you.

We typically seek psychotherapy or spirituality for the same reason: we want something to change. Not a single client has ever come to my therapy practice and said, "Glad to be here, doc. Nope, don't want to change anything. I'm good." We want something to change, but we are sometimes uncertain about what should change and how to go about changing it.

Usually, the thing we want to change is our suffering. Suffering can take many forms, including physical pain, emotional distress, and existential angst. While some suffering results from things such as illness, injury, or death, other suffering is the product of human action, such as violence, oppression, or exploitation. Wherever our suffering originates, we would prefer to suffer less and experience contentment and well-being more often. With this book comes a promise. Practice the tools and concepts in this book and you *will* experience a more consistent feeling of well-being. You will learn how to be more in control of your well-being rather than have it controlled by circumstance.

# How This Book Can Help You

One of the biggest problems people face today is the growing prevalence of mental health issues such as anxiety, depression, and stress. Despite advances in medicine and technology, rates of mental health issues continue to rise, and many people struggle to find effective and accessible solutions. This is where *The Mindful Path: Combining Psychotherapy and Buddhist Practices* comes in. This book offers an evidence-based approach to improving mental health and well-being—and to easing the suffering that has become so prevalent in our lives.

Psychology is a scientific study of human behavior and functioning and relies on observation and the scientific method to arrive at understanding and insight. Buddhist philosophy is likewise empirical, relying on the scientific method. Buddhism relies on understanding and insight gained through introspection and careful observation of direct experience. Both address why people suffer and how to ease that suffering.

Even for people who do not consider themselves "spiritual," the approach outlined in this book can still improve mental health and well-being by incorporating Buddhist practices that are thousands of years old, such as mindfulness meditation and the Eightfold Path, with evidence-based modern psychotherapy approaches, such as cognitive behavioral therapy. The techniques and methods presented here are grounded in research and proven to effectively reduce symptoms of anxiety, depression, and stress. I offer them in a secular and accessible manner, making them suitable for people of all backgrounds and beliefs.

The practices presented focus on the development of self-awareness and emotion-regulation skills. These skills benefit everyone, regardless of belief or spiritual orientation. Creating greater self-awareness and emotion-regulation skills can enable individuals to better understand their patterns of thinking and feeling, and to develop more effective coping strategies.

Here are some things to keep in mind while exploring the concepts and tools in this book:

- **Take your time:** We will cover a lot of material, and it is essential to take your time as you read each chapter. Take breaks and don't rush through the material. Allow yourself time to reflect on the material and practice the exercises before moving on to the next chapter.

- **Practice regularly:** The approaches presented in this book, such as mindfulness, meditation, or journaling, are most effective when practiced regularly. Commit to practicing these activities regularly. Even a few minutes of daily practice can improve your mental health and well-being.
- **Engage with the material:** This book includes exercises and reflection questions designed to help you engage with the material more deeply. Take the time to complete these exercises and reflect on your experiences. Consider keeping a journal to document your progress and insights.
- **Be open-minded:** The approach presented in this book combines Buddhist practices with evidence-based psychotherapy techniques. If you are new to either of these frameworks, try to hold an open mind and suspend judgments or preconceived notions. Approach the material with curiosity and a willingness to learn.
- **Seek support if needed:** While the practices presented in this book can reduce symptoms of anxiety, depression, and stress, they are not a substitute for professional help. If you are struggling with mental health issues, consider seeking support from a mental health professional.

# My Journey on the Mindful Path

When I was a young boy in middle school, I became intrigued by a television show about a young monk. The monk was the son of an American father and a Chinese mother who was orphaned at a young age and then raised in a Shaolin Monastery until he had to flee to America to escape the bounty put on his life by the Chinese emperor.

Each episode had the general format of the monk wandering around western America in the late 1800s. He usually encountered a situation that escalated into a kung fu fight with one or more bad guys. The storyline was punctuated with flashbacks of him growing up in the monastery. I was amazed at how the kind, humble, soft-spoken monk quickly subdued the bad guys. My friends and I would all be excited: "Did you see that episode last night? What'd you think when he did that spinning back kick and flipped the guy? Man, so cool."

I was less vocal about but equally interested in the lessons the young monk received from the elderly teachers in the flashback scenes in the monastery. It was nice to have the validation of my best friend, who also was intrigued by the lessons from the elder monks. (It is a good thing to have an old soul as a best friend growing up. It helps when someone understands things that are hard to put into words.) These lessons were rich in philosophies of Taoism, Confucianism, and Buddhist concepts. The influence of Buddhism on the show was particularly strong. I believe that the little pieces of wisdom I could understand at that young age were pivotal in my thinking and helped me to cope effectively in middle school and onward.

The monk in the show usually seemed calm and peaceful no matter what was going on, whether walking by himself in the woods, helping someone in need, or protecting an innocent or himself from bad guys. He often quoted Buddhist ideas and used Buddhist practices such as meditation and mindfulness to guide his actions. Over the course of watching many episodes, I came to understand that being calm, centered, and content was not a function of a particular circumstance but rather what the mind was doing. The character was a skilled martial artist but humble and compassionate, despite the suffering he experienced in his young life.

Why do people suffer? This question was often in my thoughts. I was always curious why some people seemed happy and well, and others were often angry, anxious, or sad. The question of why people suffer is complex and multifaceted. There likely is not a single answer that applies to all cases. This did not stop me from trying to find one.

Because of my persistent interest in why people suffer, I became curious about Buddhist philosophy, which is likely why I pursued a career as a clinical psychologist. In my years of practicing, I have visited with many people with varied problems. Understanding that everyone's journey is unique, I take an eclectic approach to therapy. However, I find concepts from cognitive behavioral therapy (CBT) useful for a wide variety of issues and will emphasize this framework as we explore different issues. Sometimes I listen to an individual and have a sense of their problems fitting directly into a concept from CBT; I enjoy sharing one tool or another that they could apply to address their problem. Other times, their issue brings to mind a Buddhist concept; I enjoy exploring a Buddhist idea with them, even if I don't explicitly label it as such. I gradually realized over the years that these distinct supportive interventions *together* provide a very practical framework for personal growth. Sometimes our modern psychology approach can use a boost from wisdom that has stood the test of time. Sometimes ancient wisdom can be supported with tools developed from modern scientific methods.

Keep in mind that I do not intend this book to be an in-depth treatise on Buddhism. I am not an expert on Buddhism. There are many other good academic resources for those who want to learn about this philosophy in more depth (Keown, 2004; Hanh, 1998; Gethin, 1998; Rahula, 1978; see the bibliography). For those who have never been exposed to Buddhist ideas, I hope to provide an understandable introduction to the basics of this philosophy and how it can be a helpful framework for practical self-development.

For those who have never been exposed to CBT concepts, this book is also not meant to be a CBT literature review or a compilation of techniques. It focuses on the various CBT concepts and general psychotherapy tools that people struggling with difficulties find helpful. Consider it an introduction to CBT. Many of these tools and ideas overlap significantly with the Buddhist framework of the Eightfold Path.

## The Path Forward . . .

What I offer you in this book is a compilation of concepts and techniques gathered and honed over thirty-five years of practice and visiting with hundreds of people about various issues. Many have expressed thanks for what they have learned from our sessions. What they don't always consider is how the learning is a two-way street. I have learned a great deal from them as well. They have taught me what speaks to them, what is effective, and what has been most helpful on their journey.

I hope that the insights and techniques presented in this book will be useful to you on your journey toward more significant mental health and well-being. I understand that everyone's journey is unique, and it is an honor to offer support and guidance as you navigate the challenges of modern life. My wish is for the practices and perspectives shared here to act as a valuable resource for you now and in the future. May your suffering diminish across these pages.

# Part I

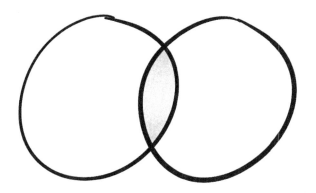

# Where Ancient Wisdom
# Meets Modern Psychology

# 1

# BUDDHISM

*Do not believe in anything simply because you have heard it. Do not believe in traditions because they have been handed down for many generations. Do not believe anything because it is spoken and rumored by many. Do not believe in anything because it is written in your religious books. Do not believe in anything merely on the authority of your teachers and elders. But after observation and analysis, when you find that anything agrees with reason and is conducive to the good and the benefit of one and all, then accept it and live up to it.*

*– The Buddha*

# Who Was the Buddha?

According to legend, the founder of Buddhism, Siddhartha Gautama, was a historical figure born circa 563 BCE into a wealthy family. He experienced a life of riches and comfort, and he was shielded from the suffering of those outside the palace walls. Disgruntled by his lack of knowledge of his subjects, one day he quietly ventured outside his gilded haven. There he saw the suffering of the poor, illness, old age, and death. This contrast with his shielded life of privilege caused him to experience an existential crisis. How could he be delighted with his abundant riches and comfort, knowing there was so much suffering in the world?

Dissatisfied with a life of fleeting pleasures, he sought a more profound truth to better understand the human condition, and he embraced a lifestyle of asceticism or extreme self-discipline. Asceticism was a dominant spiritual practice at the time. Ascetics believe that enlightenment comes from renouncing all worldly pleasures. After several years of practicing various forms of severe self-deprivation, he realized these practices did not seem to hold the answers he sought. Neither the comfort of self-indulgence nor the extreme discipline of self-denial seemed to lead to answers to his questions about human suffering. Siddhartha then resolved to meditate until he had either died or gained full enlightenment.

After sitting under a tree for many days and nights and mindfully enduring distractions, he experienced total clarity and insight. After several weeks spent processing this moment and debating his ability to effectively share his realization with others, he taught the first of several sermons in which he expounded the Four Noble Truths and the Eightfold Path. From then on, he became known as the Buddha. Buddha is a Sanskrit word for *enlightened one*.

It is important to note that the Buddha is not a deity. He is just a human being who developed essential insights into the human condition. In this sense, Buddhism is not a religion in the traditional sense but more like a philosophy or way of life. *After careful observation and introspection, this is what we have observed. What have you observed from your direct experience?*

Buddhism has no "creed" that one must accept to be on team Buddha. Instead, one is asked to rely on feedback from direct experience. What does your direct experience tell you vs. what I tell you? Buddhism is described as "a way of life" (Rahula, 1978, p. 81), and there are no external rites or ceremonies to follow to become Buddhist. One merely needs to understand and practice the Buddha's teachings. One author has explained that the Buddha teaches an attitude rather than an affiliation, and that this state of mind can be acquired by any ordinary individual willing to put in the practice (Khong, 2003). "Each individual can develop this attitude through self-discovery and self-understanding, a process that calls for personal responsibility and effort rather than affiliation" (p. 72).

# The Middle Way

One of the Buddha's first realizations was that suffering seems to derive from extremes. The middle path refers to avoiding two extremes of everyday life: indulgence in sensual pleasures on the one hand and severe asceticism on the other. He cautioned that one could become attached to sensual indulgence and self-denial. Instead, he describes a way, or path, that transcends and reconciles the duality that characterizes most thinking.

Seeking pleasure and indulging in worldly desires does not free us from suffering. When one desire is met, others spring up, leaving us in a perpetual state of wanting. But this doesn't mean we should gravitate to the opposite extreme. We don't have to reject all worldly experiences to attain peace. Attempting to do so is exhausting and keeps us in inner conflict. Every day, we need comfort, food, and connection with others. The Buddha's insight was that the ascetic path leaves us averse to the everyday experiences of life. Being averse to the normal experience of life attaches us to the suffering we are trying to diminish.

The Middle Way offers a balanced approach. The Buddha found the answer he sought by taking the middle position between indulgence and self-denial. The way to free oneself from suffering is to be as centered as possible in that balanced, contented state which is neither self-denial nor desire.

It is part of being human to desire things. To pretend we don't have desire goes against our nature, creating inner conflict. We might suppress it for a while, but the suppression usually won't last indefinitely. Even if we could successfully stop a specific desire, another would soon arise.

On the other hand, even if you figure out a way to get what you want, your happy state also doesn't last. Soon, a desire for something else arises. The satisfaction you received from fulfilling your desire fades, and having what you want no longer eases your suffering. When we occupy the Middle Way, we can experience desire without getting consumed or preoccupied. When we notice that desire rises and dissipates, we realize it's momentary. You don't have to fulfill all desires or reject them. Because you haven't taken them too seriously, you're free from desire.

On the other end of the spectrum, we find the opposite of desire: aversion. Aversion reflects our attempts to avoid suffering by avoiding unpleasant experiences or emotions. Ironically, trying to avoid suffering brings about suffering. When we don't want to experience something unpleasant, emotions such as anxiety, fear, anger, or disgust arise. Ram Dass reminds us: "The resistance to the unpleasant situation is the root of suffering."

The Middle Way's solution to aversion is the same as its solution to desire. We face it from the middle position. We don't indulge our aversions by running away from what we dislike. Nor do we attempt to renounce our aversions by rejecting their existence or deeming what we dislike to be wrong or bad. Instead, we acknowledge our tendencies toward aversion as part of human nature and learn to move through them skillfully. Remaining centered in the middle position, we can experience the discomfort of anxiety, anger, fear, or disgust that arises around what we view as unpleasant.

The more we practice creating a space for uncomfortable sensations and emotions to rise and fall—without acting on them—the more they lose their grip on us. Anxiety and anger push us to *do something*. I must do something to make the feeling go away. We discover we can learn to tolerate the discomfort of unpleasant experiences without doing anything. We accept that they are an undeniable part of the human experience, and that our resistance to them prolongs and increases our suffering.

In Buddhist practice, striving with determination refers to putting in effort toward achieving a specific goal, such as a peaceful mind. Conversely, equanimity refers to remaining calm and composed when facing either success or failure and not being overly attached to the outcome. Striving with determination is an essential aspect of Buddhist practice, as effort and discipline are necessary to overcome obstacles and achieve one's goals. Equanimity, on the other hand, helps to prevent attachment and aversion, which can lead to suffering.

There are several ways we practice the Middle Way in everyday life. For example, the Middle Way in diet entails avoiding overeating and under-eating, and instead consuming food in moderation. This means not indulging in unhealthy foods but also not depriving oneself of necessary nutrition. The Middle Way in work-life balance means neither overworking nor under-working. This involves finding a sustainable pace that allows for both productivity and relaxation. In relationships, the Middle Way means avoiding both attachment and aversion. This involves cultivating a sense of detachment and equanimity toward others while practicing compassion and loving-kindness. In general, the practice entails avoiding both excessive devotion and neglect. This means balancing study and practice of the Buddha's teachings (dharma) with being mindful of daily life activities.

The Middle Way is not a tepid compromise between two extremes, but a balanced and holistic approach to life. It is not about finding a midpoint between two opposing views, but rather recognizing the limitations and suffering associated with clinging to either extreme.

The Middle Way considers impermanence to be a fundamental aspect of reality. It acknowledges that everything, including all phenomena and experiences, constantly changes. To overcome our attachment and aversion, it encourages us to recognize the fundamental truth of impermanence. By acknowledging and accepting that everything is transient and subject to change, we can learn to let go of our clinging or resistance to something that ultimately brings suffering.

The Middle Way also emphasizes the importance of finding a balance between being present in the moment and planning for the future. Even though everything is impermanent and subject to change, we still need to plan and prepare for the future while remaining mindful and present in the current moment.

## The Four Noble Truths

According to traditional accounts of Buddhism, the Buddha's first sermon, known as "Setting in Motion the Wheel of Dharma," focused on the Four Noble Truths. While the Middle Way is a central teaching in many Buddhist traditions, the Buddha did not introduce it in his first sermon. However, it is typically understood as a complementary teaching to the Four Noble Truths rather than a replacement for them.

The *First Noble Truth* is that there is suffering in life. This observation is better than it sounds. The English translation of the Sanskrit word *dukkha* is "suffering." Some scholars say the word is perhaps better defined as "incapable of satisfying." Other scholars translate *dukkha* as "stressful."

Everything is impermanent. Conditions change, and we suffer when attached to how they used to be. We experience happiness, but that too is impermanent and changes, so we suffer when our happiness does not last. This first truth helps us understand that life is unsatisfying because nothing lasts. We live in bodies that constantly want things to maintain a balance, making us suffer because balance also is impermanent. The Buddha's observation was that *dukkha* seems inescapable when we try to deny or escape this reality that creates more suffering. *Why am I suffering? I shouldn't be suffering.* Now I suffer from not wanting to suffer. We want to find that safe place where we will be permanently comfortable and life will be permanently predictable.

The *Second Noble Truth* is that there is a cause for the arising of suffering. If we look deeply at our suffering, we recognize how our actions, or lack of actions, contribute to our suffering. There is the inevitable pain that results from a fragile and impermanent life. The second truth addresses the extra pain that arises from struggling with the first truth rather than accepting its reality. It helps us to understand and look at the causes of our suffering instead of viewing it as something that randomly visits us and is therefore beyond our control. Resistance to the reality of life is the engine of our suffering. The static idea I have about who I am (*ego*) clings on the one hand and resists reality on the other. Much of the energy at the root of suffering is servicing my ego, no matter the reality before me.

The Second Noble Truth teaches that the cause of suffering is desire, or wanting and clinging to things that have changed. More precisely, it is wanting what is not possible at that moment. The word from the early writings is *tanha*, which often translates as "thirst" or "craving." If I want what is possible, then moving toward what I want is simple. *I am thirsty, so I will pour myself a glass of water.* Simple. But what if I am where there is no water, and I am thirsty, AND I really want something to drink (even though that is not possible at that moment)? Now I am suffering from being thirsty. Before, I was merely thirsty. But now, because I *want* something to drink when I am in a situation that doesn't allow me to get something to drink, I am *suffering* from thirst. Thirst alone is not suffering. Wanting to ease the thirst and being unable to—that is suffering.

We continually search for things outside ourselves to make us happy. Even if we are very successful, we never are permanently satisfied. Even if I am fortunate to have satisfied most of my desires, the satisfaction is temporary. The second truth does not tell us to give up everything to find happiness. The actual issue here is more subtle; the *attachment* to what we desire is the problem. Our mind becomes attached and clings when it cannot accept what is true.

The Buddha taught that desire derives from ignorance of the self. Sometimes my sense of myself or *ego* gets attached to things. We attach to ideas about ourselves and the world around us. We are then frustrated when the world doesn't function the way we think it should. We don't like it when the universe does not bend to our will. Our actions can be detached from the reality of the situation when we do things to serve our ego instead of our well-being and the well-being of others. When I am preoccupied with who I am (ego, identity), I will probably focus on actions that reinforce or repair this notion. When I am busy doing this, I am not as likely to pay attention to my actions and how they affect my well-being and those around me.

The *Third Noble Truth* is that it is possible to cease suffering by not doing the things that create suffering. One way to think of the Four Noble Truths is that they are analogous to a physician diagnosing an illness and prescribing a treatment. The first truth tells us what the illness is. The second truth tells us what causes the illness. The Third Noble Truth tells us not to worry; the illness has a cure. The Third Truth teaches us that a peaceful mind is not dependent on external circumstances.

The solution to *dukkha* is to stop desire and clinging. Just stop! But how do we do that? Much easier said than done. It's impossible to tell yourself that now you will crave nothing. This doesn't work because the conditions that give rise to craving will remain present. Things will still change. We will still exist in bodies that need water and food. Things that make us happy will change and fade. The Second Noble Truth tells us that when we attach to things we believe will make us happy or give us a sense of security, they inevitably change, and then we experience suffering. Grasping for all these different things never satisfies us for long because it is all impermanent. When we understand this, we can let go of attachment. When we know this viscerally, letting go is easy. The craving will seem to disappear on its own. The Buddha taught that through practice, we could end cravings. We don't eliminate all desires, but we learn how to relate to our desires differently. But how to practice?

The *Fourth Noble Truth* is the understanding that there is a path that leads to refraining from what makes us suffer and cultivates a peaceful mind. This path of practice is called the Eightfold Path. The First Noble Truth defines the illness, which is suffering. The Second Noble Truth tells us that the illness has a cause. The Third Noble Truth, by addressing the cause, tells us we can cure the illness. Finally, the Fourth Noble Truth is the prescription to address the cause of the illness.

# The Eightfold Path

The Eightfold Path comprises eight interrelated practices:

- Right Understanding
- Right Thought
- Right Speech
- Right Action
- Right Livelihood
- Right Effort
- Right Concentration
- Right Mindfulness

In this context, the word "right" does not refer to a moral judgment, but an empirical one. For example, there are straightforward, beneficial ways to practice mindfulness. Wrong mindfulness would mean ways of practice that are not beneficial. Someone does not impose arbitrarily right and wrong from the outside. You can look to your own experience and answer the question for yourself: is this beneficial ("right") or not helpful ("wrong")? Sometimes the original Pali word is translated as wise. Some have noted that the English translation can feel judgmental: Right vs. Wrong, Wise vs. Foolish. One writer has suggested the word "spacious" (Noble, 2011). *Right* has a sense of being beneficial, skillful, reducing suffering, wholesome, and in alignment with reality. *Wrong*, not so much. What *works* to bring about a positive result? Is this the "right" key to unlock and open the door?

Think about the set of keys you carry with you wherever you go. A key helps us to move beyond a barrier of some sort. If we have the "right" key, the door opens and we can then enter the space. Use the "wrong" key, and the door won't open and the space is not available to us. This is what is meant by "right" for the distinct elements of the Eightfold Path. Am I using the "right" approach that will open the space of a peaceful mind?

The eight aspects of the Path are not followed and practiced one after another in numerical order. The Path refers to practicing these eight interconnected aspects daily as you move through your life. Each supports the practice of the others. The practice is keeping all eight aspects in mind as much as possible.

These eight factors aim at promoting and perfecting the three essentials of Buddhist training and discipline: *wisdom, ethical conduct,* and *mental discipline.* Wisdom reflects the practice of Right View and Right Thought. Wisdom is seeing things as they are and having thoughts aligned with this view of reality. If we see things as they are, and have thoughts aligned with reality, we have a greater sense of well-being than if we twist reality in a way that deviates from how things are.

Ethical conduct reflects this wisdom in the practice of Right Action, Right Speech, and Right Livelihood. Again, ethical conduct in this context is more than just a list of rules. It is the idea that when we conduct ourselves ethically with others, such as in our actions, speech, and how we make a living, it facilitates a more peaceful way of being. Keeping a concentrated focus on these things requires mental discipline. Mental discipline includes the practice of Right Effort, Right Mindfulness, and Right Concentration. Practicing the path requires appropriate effort, being mindful of our understanding, thoughts, and actions, and maintaining focus when necessary.

And how do we walk this noble path? The idea is not to follow assertions in some abstract or dogmatic philosophical perspective, but rather a very practical one. Walking the Path means being disciplined in applying these ideas in our everyday life.

For some folks, the word discipline can feel oppressive. It implies a grimly focused person who has no fun. It can beg the question— why not just follow my passions and focus all my effort on pursuing and gaining whatever makes me happy? Why should I impose discipline when life is already such a struggle? However, in the Buddhist sense, discipline is not some joyless drudgery. It represents a pragmatic middle path that avoids extremes and serves as a practice to keep us on a path of cultivating well-being in ourselves and others, rather than giving in to our natural impulses to fall into suffering.

The practice is like a two-sided coin, in that a person must equally develop two connected qualities. These qualities are compassion and wisdom. It is much like a bird needing two wings to fly. Compassion represents love, kindness, tolerance, charity, and other similar qualities of emotion or the heart. Wisdom stands for the intellectual side, or the qualities of the mind. "If one develops only the emotional, neglecting the intellectual, one may become a good-hearted fool. To develop only the intellectual side and neglect the emotional may turn one into a hard-hearted intellect without feeling for others. Therefore, one must develop both equally to be balanced and content" (Rahula, 1978).

The Eightfold Path is also best thought of as a practice. It is not like a light switch that I turn on, and now I understand all. It is a framework for practice. We become good at what we practice. If we practice bad habits, we get good at them. If we practice things that support well-being in ourselves and others, we will also get good at those.

In this context, I like the word "cultivate." Developing a peaceful mind is very much like tending to a garden. You first must decide what you want to grow. You must prepare the soil to receive the seeds you want to sow. You must be attentive, water the garden, and provide fertilizer so the roots can develop and grow into seedlings. During this early process, weeds may overtake the fragile seedlings you are trying to grow. You must pull out the weeds by their roots before they overtake what you intend to grow.

Over time, the plant becomes strong and develops deep roots. If you do all this, you will have a functional garden. However, if you turn away and ignore what is growing in your garden, you may come back and notice that weeds are overtaking everything. This intentional process applies also when trying to develop a peaceful mind. You are not waiting passively for the fairies to deliver to you a functional garden; you are preparing the ground and tending the plants you want to grow.

## The Path Forward . . .

In this chapter, we explored some basic ideas of Buddhism. We learned that the Buddha was not a deity, just a regular guy who struggled with the question of suffering like most of us. Through careful introspection, he understood some fundamental truths about the human experience. He realized that much of suffering comes from the extremes and that contentment is enhanced by finding the Middle Way. He realized that suffering seems to be a part of life because of the way we are made as human beings. However, he also realized that we enhance our suffering when we resist this simple truth.

Suffering has a cause, and by addressing the causes of suffering, we can enhance our well-being. The way to do this is through what he termed the Eightfold Path. The path forward is a practice, much like cultivating a garden.

Take a moment to reflect on the information presented in this chapter. What idea(s) resonated with you? Could you relate some aspect of your own suffering to these concepts?

In the next chapter, we will explore the basics of cognitive behavioral therapy. While reading about the basics of this approach, try to notice similarities with the Buddhist ideas explored so far.

# 2

# COGNITIVE BEHAVIORAL THERAPY (CBT)

*"If our thinking is bogged down by distorted symbolic meanings,*
*illogical reasoning and erroneous interpretations,*
*we become, in truth, blind and deaf".*
*–Aaron Beck*

Cognitive behavioral therapy (CBT) is a type of therapy that involves identifying and challenging unhelpful thoughts and behaviors. In this therapy, you learn alternative thinking patterns and behaviors, which can improve your emotions. Much like a Buddhist framework, CBT involves understanding basic concepts and then practicing applying them to change thoughts and behaviors that are causing stress and undermining one's well-being. CBT evolved from two schools of psychology: behaviorism and cognitive therapy.

Behavioral treatment for mental disorders has been around since the early 1900s. Behaviorism is based on the idea that behaviors can be measured, modeled, and changed with techniques such as positive reinforcement or systematic exposure. Behavioral therapy gained prominence in the 1940s in response to the emotional difficulties faced by veterans returning from war. This need for effective short-term treatment for depression and anxiety coincided with behavioral research regarding how people learn to behave and react to life situations. Behaviorism offered an alternative to the dominant model of that time, psychoanalysis. Two psychologists in the 1950s and 1960s spurred the development of cognitive therapy.

American psychologist Albert Ellis was a key figure who stressed the importance of thoughts, feelings, and behaviors and devised a theory called rational emotive behavior therapy (REBT) in the 1950s. This early form of cognitive psychotherapy was based on the idea that a person's negative emotions or stress arise from their thoughts about an event rather than the actual event itself. In this framework, the goal is to change irrational beliefs to more rational ones, thereby changing the negative emotions associated with irrational beliefs. REBT encourages people to identify their irrational beliefs (e.g., *I must be perfect, I'm a failure, everything is hopeless*) and then coaches them to challenge and correct these false beliefs. In this sense, it is very similar to the Buddhist concept of suffering deriving from thoughts not in alignment with Right Understanding.

Ellis (1962) proposed that each of us holds a unique set of assumptions about ourselves as well as our world around us. These assumptions guide us through life and determine our reactions to the various situations we encounter. Some assumptions are irrational and lead us to perpetuate negative mood states. He called these beliefs *basic irrational assumptions*. For example, some people irrationally assume that they are a failure if they do not succeed at everything they attempt to do. This assumption affects all their interactions, so even a minor setback can leave them dissatisfied and feeling like a failure despite all other accomplishments.

Ellis noted other common irrational assumptions:
* People have no control over their happiness.
* One should be thoroughly competent at everything.
* It is catastrophic when things are not how you want them to be.
* You need someone stronger than yourself to depend on.
* Your history greatly influences your present life.
* There is a solution to every human problem, and it's a disaster if you don't find it.

In the 1960s, another psychologist, Aaron Beck, noticed patterns in the thinking of his depressed clients. These patients held a negative view of themselves, others, and their future. In therapy, they would hold on to these beliefs no matter how much exploration of their past occurred. Exploration of history was the predominant form of psychotherapy at the time, usually based on Freudian psychological theories. This led Beck to research whether holding negative views about self, others, and the world might be a significant reason people become depressed (Beck, 1967).

Beck identified three factors that he thought were responsible for depression:

1. The cognitive triad (of automatic negative thinking)
2. Negative self-schemas
3. Errors in logic (i.e., faulty information processing)

The cognitive triad reflects three interrelated forms of negative thinking that are typical of individuals with depression: negative thoughts about the self (*I'm a failure. I'm worthless and undesirable*), the world (*Nobody cares for me. Things are stacked against me*) and the future (*Nothing I do matters, so why even try? It's always going to be this way*).

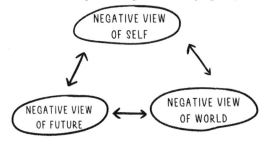

These three components interact and interfere with normal cognitive processing, leading to distorted perceptions, selective memory, and poor problem-solving. The person holding these negative thoughts repeatedly has their efforts to cultivate peace or well-being undermined.

Butler and Beck (2000) reviewed fourteen meta analyses[1] to explore the effectiveness of Beck's cognitive therapy. They concluded that about eighty percent of adults benefited from it. They also found that cognitive therapy was more successful than drug therapy and had a lower relapse rate. This finding supported the proposition that depression has a cognitive component. Cognitive therapy is effective with a wide range of issues, such as depression, anxiety, sexual disorders, eating disorders, insomnia, and substance abuse, and even as an adjunctive treatment for major psychiatric disorders such as bipolar disorder or schizophrenia.

Behavioral therapies have been successful in treating several conditions, including phobias and anxiety. As the popularity of cognitive therapies has soared, therapists have incorporated behavioral techniques to treat disorders successfully. Although behavioral and cognitive schools of thought have different emphases, both are concerned with what is happening to the individual in the present rather than exploring historical factors. Integrating behavioral and cognitive therapies became known as cognitive behavioral therapy (CBT).

The core principles of CBT are that psychological problems are based partly on faulty or unhelpful ways of thinking. They are also a result of learned patterns of unhelpful behavior and coping mechanisms. CBT has showed that people suffering from psychological problems can learn tools to change thinking and behavior patterns and cope skillfully.

In CBT, you first learn to recognize thought patterns and internal narratives related to negative mood states, stress, and the sense of self. The next step is to apply tools to challenge and change these ways of looking at things. It is a study of how your perceptions affect your emotions.

CBT teaches you to recognize behavioral patterns and try new, more adaptive behaviors. Some concepts may seem counterintuitive. For example,

---

1    *A meta-analysis is an advanced statistical technique that combines the results of multiple studies that look at similar questions. It is the gold standard of summarizing the academic research in an area.*

anxiety makes us prone to try to escape or avoid, while moving toward, rather than away, is in fact the means for overcoming anxiety. If the moving toward is done correctly, anxiety is diminished. Sometimes a particular coping pattern that relieves us of stress in the short term can cause more stress in the long term.

A great deal of research provides empirical support for the effectiveness of CBT methods. CBT also is empirically based at the level of individual therapy. The person using the tools will test out beliefs in various ways to determine if they align with the situation or are distorted. They will then try new behaviors and observe the resultant effect on their emotions.

# Overlap of Buddhism and CBT

Buddhism and CBT are both systematic explorations of suffering. Why am I stressed? Why am I sad? What factors give rise to my suffering? Both systems are focused on this fundamental question of suffering. Both systems have an insight that suffering is common to the human condition. Both also see that suffering has a cause, and by examining what is contributing to our suffering and changing those conditions, we can reduce our suffering and improve the sense of well-being in ourselves as well as others.

The CBT framework and the Middle Way support a balanced and practical approach to life, as they emphasize finding a balanced perspective and avoiding extreme thoughts or behaviors. CBT encourages individuals to find a middle ground between opposing thoughts or emotions and to develop more balanced and rational thinking patterns. Individuals can reduce their symptoms and improve their overall well-being by finding a more balanced perspective and avoiding black-and-white thinking.

Buddhism also takes an empirical approach to the study of suffering. Buddhism does not have a creed, per se. It simply articulates an understanding based on careful study and introspection. You are not required to "believe" in a particular understanding. It is more like: "This is what we have observed. What does your direct experience tell you when you examine it carefully?" CBT has a very similar empirical approach. It doesn't assert "beliefs," but instead employs the scientific method. "This is our best understanding based on the research. Now, let's test this understanding under various conditions and see how it holds up." As we use the scientific method, our understanding gets increasingly refined. The application of research in a clinical setting takes the same empirical approach.

"Let's try this tool, see how it works based on your experience, then change it as necessary." Like the Buddhist path, CBT is not an approach that relies on simply "understanding" CBT concepts. To be effective, we must practice the concepts. Remember, *we get good at what we practice.*

While these two approaches may seem very different, they share many fundamental principles that can be integrated helpfully. CBT and Buddhism strongly emphasize the relationship between thoughts, emotions, and behaviors, recognizing that our thoughts and beliefs can have a powerful impact on our mental and emotional well-being. CBT seeks to help individuals identify and challenge negative or irrational thought patterns. Buddhism teaches that we can train the mind to cultivate positive states of consciousness and reduce suffering.

Buddhism emphasizes the importance of cultivating mindfulness, compassion, and self-awareness, which are also central values in CBT. By integrating mindfulness and compassion practices into CBT, individuals can deepen their understanding of their thought patterns and emotions and develop a greater sense of inner calm and resilience.

Another similarity between these two approaches is the focus on taking action to ease suffering. Buddhism involves following the Eightfold Path and engaging in activities committed to compassion and non-harm. CBT uses specific techniques to change negative thoughts and behaviors and develop new, more adaptive coping skills. It is essential to do the work to make effective changes actively. The movement from suffering to well-being is an active practice in both frameworks.

Integrating CBT and Buddhism can offer a comprehensive and practical approach to promoting mental and emotional well-being. By combining the valuable tools and techniques of CBT with the wisdom and compassion of Buddhism, individuals can cultivate a greater sense of self-awareness, develop healthier thought patterns, and find greater peace and happiness.

## The Path Forward . . .

Modern psychology, like Buddhism, explores the basic question of why people suffer. Cognitive behavioral therapy (CBT) is a particular area of modern psychology that has explored, through the scientific method, why people suffer. This approach has been well researched and is very effective in helping people deal with their suffering.

Take a moment to reflect on the concepts in this chapter. Have you noticed a connections between your thinking patterns and your feelings? What ideas do take as a given that might be a source of suffering for you? What behaviors do you repeatedly engage in that might contribute to your suffering?

In the following chapters, I will present an introductory understanding of each aspect of the Eightfold Path. We will then explore CBT concepts or tools that reflect and support the Buddhist framework. Much like CBT, Buddhism does not insist you merely believe in the Eightfold Path. It is a practice of viewing things differently and doing things differently. As we explore the Eightfold Path, incorporating CBT concepts that fit within the eight interrelated practices, we will start with concepts from ancient wisdom and then give the ancient wisdom a boost from modern psychology.

# Part II

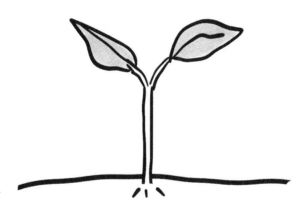

# *Cultivating Wisdom*

# 3

# RIGHT UNDERSTANDING

*"Everything that has a beginning has an end.
Make your peace with that, and all will be well."
–Buddha*

# Buddhism and Right Understanding

Right Understanding is based on the idea of seeing things as they are. It is acceptance of certain aspects of reality that are sometimes difficult to accept. It is challenging to understand that things are temporary and that, many times, our wants are not possible right now. Right Understanding is being aware of our limits as human beings. It is mindful of difficulties presented by perception. Right Understanding is based on acceptance, seeing life as it is. It aligned with reality. Buddhist philosophy has ideas about Right Understanding. CBT also teaches concepts about how reality seems to operate. Being in alignment with this understanding leads to fewer problems and stress.

## Understanding Impermanence

One of the core concepts of Buddhist philosophy is the idea of impermanence. Nothing lasts forever, and everything changes. Our thoughts, feelings, bodies, and the world around us continuously change. Even our views change over time as we consider things from different angles. We learn new things and forget other things. We like the illusion of permanence because it gives us a sense of security. We become attached to this feeling of security and become distressed when the inevitable reality of impermanence intrudes. We enjoy our pleasures and feel a sense of loss when they fade. We fear times of difficulty because we suspect they may be permanent. Because everything is impermanent and nothing lasts, nothing can be held onto. Our minds attach to things as though they are static when, in fact, everything is continuously changing.

Impermanence is life's number one inescapable and essentially painful fact. It is the basic existential problem that the Buddhist practice addresses. We are ever-changing, like the weather. Understanding impermanence is at the deepest core of the Buddhist path. The Buddha's last words express this: *Impermanence is inescapable. Everything vanishes.*

We can intellectually appreciate the idea of impermanence. *Yes, I know, eventually, my shoes wear out.* However, emotionally we feel uneasy when we think about impermanence. During my typical day, I expect most things to be as they were yesterday. I am shocked or upset on occasions when reality intrudes, and something changes. *Every day for the last four years, my car started when I turned the key. Today it did not.* When this happens, I have an uneasy feeling coupled perhaps with feelings of sadness, anger, or fear.

The loss aspect of impermanence seems depressing at first glance. If everything vanishes eventually, then what's the point? However, impermanence is also change. Difficult situations can change. Change can be growth or renewal. Change, even when sought after, provokes a mixture of feelings. If something new emerges, something old is lost. Even this unpleasant status of the present is not permanent.

Once we understand impermanence and practice awareness of this reality, our approach to daily life is lighter and more fluid. We no longer hold on to things as though they are static. Our minds are not colliding with reality, but are flexibly aligned with it. We can more easily let go of attachments to people, objects, or situations, as we recognize they will inevitably change or pass away.

Impermanence can help us accept changes in our relationships, career, possessions, and health. By recognizing that change is inevitable, we can learn to accept and adapt to it more easily. It can also remind us that the present moment is all we have, as the past is gone and the future is uncertain. This can encourage us to be more mindful and present in our daily lives, appreciating and savoring the moment.

Impermanence can also help us cope with the loss of loved ones or other significant changes. By recognizing that everything is subject to change, we can find comfort in knowing that all things, including our pain and suffering, are impermanent. It can also help us appreciate the beauty and richness of life, as we recognize everything is fleeting and precious. This can encourage us to cultivate a sense of gratitude for the people and experiences in our lives, appreciating them while we have them. Overall, impermanence can be a helpful tool for cultivating wisdom, compassion, and a sense of presence and appreciation.

Japanese cherry blossom, or *Sakura*, symbolizes impermanence in Japanese culture. The cherry blossom is a beautiful flower that blooms briefly each year. The Japanese celebrate the blooming of the cherry blossom with festivals and parties, and it is seen as a reminder of the brief nature of life. Cherry blossoms have a lifespan of typically only a week or two. Their short lifespan is a metaphor for the impermanence of all things. It reminds us that everything in life is subject to change, and that even the most beautiful and precious things will eventually pass away.

In Japanese culture, the cherry blossom is also associated with the concept of *mono no aware*, which refers to the bittersweet feeling of appreciating the impermanence and transience of life. This feeling is often expressed in Japanese literature and art, and it reflects a deep appreciation for the fleeting nature of all things, including life itself. Overall, the Japanese cherry blossom symbolizes impermanence by reminding us of the beauty and transience of life and encouraging us to appreciate the present moment while it lasts.

# Understanding the Three Poisons: Desire, Aversion, and Ignorance

In Buddhist philosophy, *desire, aversion,* and *ignorance* (sometimes called greed, hatred, and delusion) are the three poisons. The notion of a "poison" emphasizes how dangerous specific thoughts and emotions can be if they are not understood and transformed. Desire refers to our selfishness, greed, attachment, and grasping for happiness and satisfaction in the world outside of ourselves. Aversion refers to our anger and hatred toward other people, circumstances, and even toward our discomfort. Ignorance refers to our misperceptions and wrong views of reality. These poisonous states of mind then drive unskillful thoughts, speech, and actions, which cause suffering and unhappiness for ourselves and others.

Desire, aversion, and ignorance are deeply embedded in our conditioning. Buried deep in our minds, these three poisons consistently influence and corrupt our behavior. When we understand this, we can see the factors causing suffering. We can choose to eliminate them and their influence on our minds and behavior. The Four Noble Truths teach us that when we understand the exact causes of our suffering, we can take the steps to extinguish those causes.

## Desire
Our propensity to desire creates in us a burning, unquenchable thirst of sorts. The poison of desire generates an inner longing that makes us believe that if we merely get what we want, our hunger will be satisfied. We mistakenly think our happiness depends on satisfying that hunger, but once we attain it, we get no lasting satisfaction. A serious impediment to well-being is the idea that *I will be happy just as soon as* . . . Another question to ask oneself is *Why am I not happy today?* Even if we arrive at our goal, once again, desire will arise. When our minds are dominated by greed, we are never content. We get the new car and are happy, but gradually the fresh car smell and the satisfaction fade.

Another aspect of desire is a lack of generosity and compassion toward others and sometimes ourselves. We always seem to want more; we want bigger and better to fulfill our insatiable inner desires. We are attached to things and to what we think will make us happy, which often leads to a tunnel vision that makes it hard to see the suffering of others or to give resources or time to others. Our greed can fuel jealousy.

We want what the other has. Harshly judging ourselves for not having more can trigger desire. When we are in tunnel vision, our actions often are not skillful, and we hurt those close to us. This endless and pernicious cycle continues to bring suffering and unhappiness. Desire is primarily at the root of suffering when directed toward what is not possible now.

Sometimes our desires get intertwined with our egos. I want things, and when I get them, I attach some significance to my sense of who I am (ego). Having that big house or new car means I am more successful or talented than others. Go me! However, the efforts to maintain the ego can be endless and relentless because there is no lasting satisfaction. Once again, I long for a bigger house and a better car.

### Aversion

The symptoms of aversion can show up as anger, hostility, hatred, dislike, or ill-will, wishing harm or suffering upon another person. While desire is suffering that comes from longing toward things, hatred is when we habitually resist, deny, and avoid unpleasant feelings, circumstances, and people we dislike. Desire is longing for, while aversion is pushing away.

A particular suffering comes from trying to avoid suffering. We want everything to be pleasant, comfortable, and easy all the time. However, things are not statically that way. When we are averse to things, we have thoughts like *I hate it when people act that way. I hate it when it rains on me. It's too hot. It's too cold. That's too noisy. I hate it when there is so much traffic. I hate it when people are hating all the time. I just can't stand it when that happens.* How often do we say, "Ewww! That's disgusting!"? When dominated by aversion, we are caught in a perpetual mental state of being in judgment: judging other people, situations, and our own feelings. When I look at the stream of thoughts in my mind, what percentage of them are judgmental?

Aversion thrusts us into a vicious cycle of always finding conflict and enemies everywhere. When there is conflict or perceived enemies around us, our mind is never calm. We can also create conflict within our minds when we have hatred toward our uncomfortable feelings. *I hate it when I feel* . . . With aversion, we deny, resist, and push away our feelings of fear, hurt, or inadequacy, as if those feelings were the enemy. Afflicted by the poison of aversion, we create conflict and enemies in the world and within ourselves.

Equanimity is a state of emotional stability and composure in the face of life's difficulties. It is a balance of mind that allows one to remain calm and impartial, even in challenging situations. We feel peaceful and that "it's all good." Equanimity helps to prevent attachment and aversion, which can lead to suffering. When I am attached to pleasurable experiences, I am prone to disappointment; when I am averse to unpleasant experiences, I am inclined to anger, frustration, and suffering. Equanimity allows one to see things as they are without getting caught up in likes and dislikes. It enables one to respond to situations with wisdom rather than reacting to them with emotion.

### Ignorance

Ignorance is not a lack of intelligence or capability, but the effect of a distorted state of mind. Ignorance is our wrong understanding or wrong views of reality. It is our inability to understand the nature of things free of perceptual distortions. When our minds are influenced by ignorance, we do not understand life's interdependent and impermanent nature. Instead, we view what is impermanent as stable and view ourselves as separate, permanent egos. As a result, we constantly look outside ourselves for happiness, satisfaction, and solutions to our problems. This outward searching creates even more frustration, anger, and ignorance. We do not understand how our lack of understanding causes us to engage in negative and unskillful actions that create suffering. We don't realize how our perceptions can be deceptive. Sometimes our ignorance can be willful. Instead of looking carefully at the reality of our situation, we gravitate toward things that reinforce our distorted worldview. It is more pleasant to hear what confirms our views than to listen to what might contradict the filtered reality we have created for ourselves.

In short, be aware of when you want things. We think we will finally be happy if we get what we want. The reality of our human condition does not work that way. Next, don't hate. Your judging mind causes you much more suffering than you realize. Don't hate other people, don't hate your immediate situation, and don't hate how you feel. Cultivate feelings of loving-kindness toward yourself and others. Finally, do your best to understand how reality works. When we operate in ignorance, our mind is always out of sync with reality. The more out of sync we are, the more we suffer. In straightforward terms, the three poisons are "always wanting stuff, always hating stuff, and being ignorant." Let's try not to do that.

Overcoming the three poisons requires patience, care, persistence, and deep compassion for ourselves and others. The Buddha taught us that the three poisons can be transformed. We can break the chain of suffering caused by the three poisons and live a happy, fulfilling life. We can "detoxify" from the poisons.

Over time, we can free ourselves from these unhealthy ways of thinking by practicing their opposites. Instead of feeding desires and looking for well-being outside of ourselves, we can practice letting go of attachments that reinforce our egos. Instead of hating, we can practice acceptance. Practicing acceptance does not mean that we like or approve of something. It is simply aligning with reality and resisting the reflex to judge harshly. Instead of ignorance, we can practice looking at reality squarely without distortion.

## Understanding Karma

Buddhist monk Bhante Henepola Gunaratana explains that once we understand that everything we think, say, or do is a cause, inevitably leading to some effect, we will naturally want to think, say, and do things that will lead to positive results (Gunaratana, B., 2001). We will avoid having thoughts, saying things, and doing things that will lead to negative results.

Sometimes, a naïve view of karma is viewing it as some magical force that operates in the universe. You do a bad act, like being mean to someone, and karma goes out in the universe, circles back, and delivers bad outcomes, such as spilling your coffee all over yourself. Karma is not a magical force. Karma translates as "action" or "doing" and is often referred to as the "law of cause and effect." When we do things, there is a result. The result might be good, bad, or neutral. Whatever the outcome, it attaches to the action as soon as it happens. We do things, and after we do something, we experience a result (karma). The result of the action is inescapable. It is more like a law of consequences, not a particular reward or punishment.

An important aspect of karma is intention. Karma seems to attach to intention. If we accidentally hurt someone, it does not have the same effect on our mind and future results as when we intentionally hurt someone. This is also the case when we do a positive action, but our intentions are selfish. If the intention differs from the nature of the act, the effect also differs. Another aspect of karma is the echo the act leaves in our mind. Any willful act influences our mind. The more we do an act, the more likely we are to repeat it. This is as true for beneficial acts as harmful ones.

How does karma relate to guilt? Joseph Goldstein said, "In view of karmic law, guilt is an inappropriate feeling and a rather useless burden. It simply creates more unwholesome results. Understanding karma is the basis for a straightforward development of the wisdom to know whether our actions will lead to happiness and freedom or to further suffering. When we understand this, it allows us to take responsibility for past actions with compassion, appreciating that a particular act may have been unwholesome or harmful and strongly determining not to repeat it. *Guilt is a manifestation of condemnation, wisdom, an expression of sensitivity and forgiveness*" [emphasis added] (Goldstein, 2008).

We can complicate these feelings in some circumstances. There can be an occasion where I have no bad intentions, yet I am a factor in a situation with terrible consequences. Consider an auto accident where one party has no ill will, is not doing anything illegal, and has no bad intention but causes an accident where there is a loss of life. A person in this situation might try to punish themselves by denying themselves any opportunity for happiness as penance for the happiness denied the person who died. As a result, they magnify their suffering and the suffering of those around them. This cycle continues until the person learns to have compassion for themselves.

A healthy feeling of guilt is when we know we behave in a way that is contrary to our values. This feeling of guilt is our conscience trying to nudge us back into alignment with our values. It indicates being a decent human being. An unhealthy feeling of guilt is when we feel responsible for events over which we have no control. This type of guilt comes from a variation of misdirected control. Some people are in a perpetual state of responsibility with the world's weight on their shoulders, though they have no control or influence over the events they feel guilty about. They struggle because their compassion is unbounded, and they have not come to terms with their influence being bounded.

Sometimes we get concerned about justice. Somebody does something to us that causes hurt. We want them punished. They caused us suffering, and we want them to suffer equally. We want them brought before a court or tribunal and to have justice administered to them. These are understandable thoughts we have all had at one time or another. However, what we sometimes cannot see is "cosmic justice." The idea of karma is that the effect attaches to the act when the action is done. It is inescapable. There is no need for a jury or tribunal. The "punishment," a.k.a. karma, is administered as soon as we complete the act.

# CBT and Right Understanding

## Understanding the Problem of Perception
The Buddha advised us not to be fooled by what we perceive. He said, "Where there is perception, there is deception." Thich Nhat Hanh notes that the Buddha also taught that most of our perceptions are erroneous and most of our suffering comes from wrong perceptions (Hanh, 1998).

How do we see things as they are? This is difficult because we are limited in our access to and understanding of "reality." We regularly access "reality," a filtered version of the broader, ultimate Reality. Let's examine some classic optical illusions to illustrate this point.

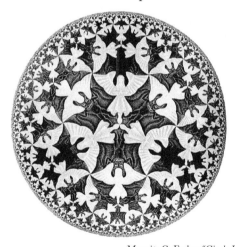

*Figure 1: Reversible figure drawing:*
*Maurits C. Escher, "Circle Limit IV (Heaven and Hell)" (Escher, 1971)*

Examine this figure. How would you describe it? Do you see bats or maybe demons? The dark space is, well, somewhat dark. Now, look closely at the white space. What do you see? You may now notice many serene angles. This figure illustrates how perception is a filtering process. We can sometimes screen out half of what we are looking at without realizing it. When we are suffering, we rarely realize how we may be selective in our perceptions. We may only perceive part of the situation. This might lead us to an unintentionally pessimistic view or a failure to see a solution to a problem.

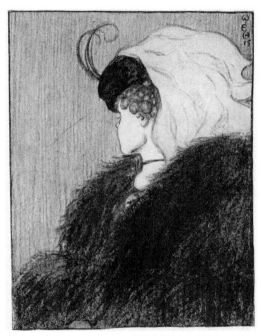

*Figure 2: Aristocrat or Witch.(Boring, 1930)*

Now examine the following figure. How would you describe the woman in the picture? Do you see a young, attractive, aristocratic-looking woman? Or do you see an older, witch-like woman? If you see the younger woman, you probably view the figure as looking away to her right. If you see the older woman, you are probably seeing her looking forward (to the viewers left) where the young woman's jawline is the old woman's nose, and the young woman's ear is the old woman's eye. What this figure illustrates is how perception is not just a passive process. When we perceive things, we actively construct the final perception. When we arrange a set of elements one way, we get a certain result. But the same elements arranged a different way in our mind gives us a different result, sometimes the exact opposite. Sometimes our perception of a situation generates suffering. If I change the way I view a situation, my suffering may change as well.

Another problem with perception is that how something appears depends on what is next to it. If I stand next to a child, I seem very tall. If I stand next to an NBA basketball player, I look short. My height remains the same, but the appearance of my height changes with the context.

This perceptual shifting of judgements about size also occurs with judgements about more abstract issues. For example, I might make a judgement about how "awful" a situation is, but my judgement will change when I compare my situation with others. So "the worst situation ever" might become "not so bad" when gauged next to losing a limb or having a serious illness.

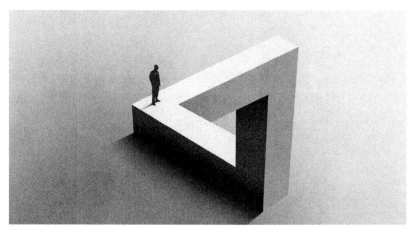

*Figure 3: Up or Down?*

So, what do these optical illusions tell us about perception? First, perception is a process of filtering what we look at. We can sometimes filter out over half of what we see and not realize it. Second, perception is an active process of constructing an impression of what we see, using the elements that have passed through the filter. What we construct can differ greatly depending on how we arrange the elements. Third, perception depends on context. Much of how we see things depends on context. What is next to what we are looking at will affect how we perceive it. Finally, often (or perhaps usually) our perceptions do not accord with reality. Thankfully, however, sometimes we can do a "test" and get closer to reality than our perceptions will allow. In chapter 3, we will explore some techniques for correcting distorted perceptions that generate suffering.

The problem of perception suggests the wisdom of adopting humility toward our perceptions. It is useful to often ask ourselves questions such as *Am I looking at this correctly? Am I missing something? Is it possible I am distorting my view because of ego or some other negative motivation?* How we look at things is essential to the practice; yet, as human beings, it is very difficult to see things clearly as they are through the haze of our limited perceptions.

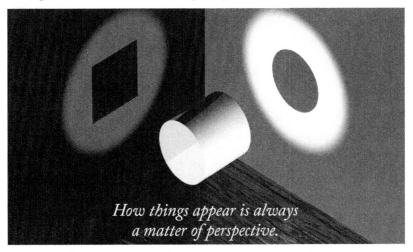

*How things appear is always a matter of perspective.*

## Understanding Imperfection

*Kintsugi* is a Japanese art of repairing broken pottery by mending the areas of breakage with lacquer mixed with gold, silver, or platinum, giving the resulting piece a unique, beautiful appearance. The philosophy behind kintsugi is that the repair is part of the history of the object, and that the cracks and breaks give the object character and beauty.

The concept of kintsugi can be viewed as a metaphor for coping with emotional or psychological trauma. Just as the broken pottery is mended and strengthened through the process of kintsugi, individuals who have experienced trauma can also learn to heal and strengthen themselves through their struggles.

The concept of kintsugi can help us understand that emotional or psychological scars are not something to be hidden or ashamed of, but something that can be embraced and celebrated as part of our unique journey. The idea that the cracks and breaks in an object can give it character and beauty can be brought to the idea that our struggles can also strengthen us and become more resilient. The songwriter Gerald

Way once said "being happy doesn't mean that everything is perfect. It means that you've decided to look beyond the imperfections."

*Wabi-sabi* is a Japanese aesthetic concept that values the beauty of things that are imperfect, impermanent, and incomplete. It is the art of finding beauty in things that are "worn," "weathered," or "aged." Wabi-sabi is often associated with Zen Buddhism and has been described as a way of living that emphasizes simplicity, humility, and the appreciation of natural and humble objects. We can learn to accept our own imperfections and impermanence. We can come to understand that these are a natural part of the human experience. This can help us develop a more accepting and compassionate view of ourselves and others, which can be beneficial for mental health and well-being.

*Turn your wounds into wisdom*
*– Oprah Winfrey*

## Understanding Subjective vs. Objective

If something is *subjective,* how it is perceived depends on the subject forming the perception. Some people like spicy food, and some do not. How do you know whether a matter is subjective or objective? If the answer depends on whom you ask, the subject is likely subjective. If something is *objective,* it doesn't change according to the subject's perception of it. For instance, 2 + 2 = 4 remains true even if you mistakenly believe 2 + 2 = 6. Opinions, preferences, and points of view are types of subjective matters. Objective matters are verifiable empirical facts.

Understanding this distinction is important, because we can make syntactical errors that can cause problems both within ourselves and in conversing with others. Consider the following sentence: "Today is Thursday." What day it happens to be is an objective fact. We can know that it is Thursday, and, if we mistakenly thought it was Friday, we could consult a resource such as a calendar and correct ourselves. I might think *I prefer to think of today as Friday,* but this preference does not change the objective fact that today is Thursday.

Now consider the next sentence "Today is a nice day." Notice how this sentence is similar in formation and sound to the previous sentence. The difference is that the subject matter is now subjective. The "niceness" of the day depends on whom you ask. Some people like brisk, cool days, and other people like warm, sunny days. However, today is Thursday, or it is not.

44

This type of syntactical error can lead to bickering with others:

*"Today is a nice day."*
*"No, it's not."*
*"Yes, it is."*
*"No, it's not. It's too cold."*
*"It's just right."*
*"No, it's not."*

And so on . . .

The problem with this dialogue is with the first statement: "Today is a nice day." This is stated as though it is a fact and anyone who disagrees is "wrong." Right and wrong do not apply to subjective matters such as preferences or opinions. Right and wrong apply to objective facts. To correct this error, we can add a *parenthetical phrase* to a statement to clarify that we are speaking from a subjective frame of reference. For example:

*Today is a nice day (for me).*
*Today is a nice day (from my point of view).*
*Today is a nice day (because I prefer cool weather over warm weather).*

There is no reason to argue for both subjective and objective matters. If you think it is Friday, and I am pretty sure it is Thursday, we should be able to appeal to a reliable source of factual information outside ourselves. If we are discussing something subjective, there is still no reason to fuss, because we are solely voicing opinions or preferences. There is no right or wrong, only different vantage points.

Often when someone has a different view, they are emphasizing a different aspect of the topic than we might emphasize:

*"I think we should buy Model A."*
*"I think we should buy Model B."*
*"From my point of view, Model A is better because it is less expensive."*
*"The way I'm looking at it, we should go with Model B because of the better quality."*

That is a simple example, but the emphasis of different aspects occurs also with more complex matters, such as the right social policy to solve a particular issue, or which religion (or nonreligion) is best. Remember that because of perception that is a complicated process. We filter out things and hence don't perceive them. We actively construct views with preferences for one thing over another. Context can significantly influence us, and sometimes we can be sure something is so even when our perceptions do not accord with reality.

These are excellent reasons for Right Understanding to include humility about our limits as human beings and how challenging it is for us to see things clearly as they are. It is often a good idea to question your perceptions and ask yourself: *Am I looking at this clearly? What am I leaving out? Is there another way I could frame this?* Over the many years I have visited with folks, those who seem to experience the most distress are those who confuse objective with subjective. They are in a world where how they see it is how it is. Such a world is rigid and unyielding. In such a world, nothing can change how they feel unless the situation changes. They think, *The universe has to bend to my will. People have to see things the way I do. My opinions are unyielding because to me they are "facts."* A bit of humility goes a long way toward being more adaptable and at peace.

## Understanding the Self: Ego vs. Action

Several modern psychological theories explore the concept of "self." One such is Self-Determination Theory, which proposes that people have innate psychological needs for autonomy, competence, and relatedness, and that fulfilling these needs leads to well-being and optimal functioning. Another is social identity theory, which states that people's sense of self is formed by their membership in social groups and the social identities associated with those groups. Self-perception theory suggests that people infer their attitudes and beliefs from their behavior and the context in which it occurs. Self-construal theory emphasizes the idea that people have different "levels" of self, including the independent self (focusing on one's own needs and goals) and the interdependent self (focusing on the needs and goals of others and one's social context). I bet you didn't think your self was so complicated!

These theories of the self in modern psychology propose that the self is a distinct, stable entity that can be understood and studied through various cognitive and social processes. In contrast, the Buddhist framework holds that the self is a fleeting, ever-changing construct that is ultimately empty of any inherent essence. What we call the self is always changing according to conditions.

One of the key differences between these perspectives is that modern psychological theories focus on the individual self as a separate entity.

Buddhism emphasizes the interconnectedness and interdependence of all things. Buddhism also stresses that attachment to the self as a permanent, unchanging entity leads to suffering, and that letting go of this attachment is critical to cultivating a feeling of well-being. Another difference is that modern psychology theories focus on the self as a cognitive and social construct. The Buddhist view focuses more on the self as a mere illusion.

Many people I visit with seem to struggle with how they view themselves. Low self-esteem is very common. Those who have experienced traumatic events often attach these experiences to some idea they have about who they are. Often the strong attachment to a framework of who they are causes a rigidity that limits their ability to change.

I used to think that the cure for "low self-esteem" was to develop "high self-esteem." By working hard at self-improvement, gaining confidence through various achievements, practicing positive affirmations, and so forth, one could learn to have a better view of oneself. However, I observed that these practices often either didn't work or the effects were short-lived or fraught with other problems.

I then came across the Buddhist concept of *anātman*, which roughly translates to *non-self*. The idea behind non-self is that there seems to be no singular, permanent thing we can define as a self. What makes up "me?" Am I my thoughts, feelings, memories, or knowledge? Am I my roles of father, spouse, friend, psychologist?

### What Is an Ego?

A self that is viewed as a permanent, unchanging thing is called the *ego*. The ego does not refer to arrogance, as in "that person has a big ego." In this context, the ego refers to ways in which we think about ourselves as having permanent, fixed characteristics or traits. If not careful, we can get into the habit of taking experiences that come and go as a permanent part of our ego. For example, if I experience a disappointing failure, I might take that transient experience and view myself as a permanent loser. Or if I experienced repeated mistreatment while growing up, I may attach those experiences to my ego and see my adult self as unlovable. The more we attach experiences to our definition of self, or ego, the more elaborate and complicated it becomes. The problem is that none of the components that make up "me" are permanent, unchanging traits. If I think otherwise, it is because of an illusion. I might suffer from low self-esteem, but if I look deeply at what "self" means, it can be puzzling to decide what it means that I dislike my "self."

When contemplating the self, we often start with the mistake of imagining some static "thing" that is persistent or permanent. We think of it as permanent despite changing conditions. So, we often ask ourselves: *Who am I?* It is natural then to answer the question with *I'm this* or *I'm that.* Then follows the natural question *Is that adequate or not?* or *Is that good enough or not?* These questions measure the ego. If my ego is some kind of permanent thing, I should be able to measure it along different dimensions and get an idea of whether it is adequate.

It is an interesting exercise to consider what your ego is. *Where is my ego? Who am I? What dimensions make up an ego?*

- **Is it in your name?** The answer is no. People could call you different names, which would not influence your being.
- **Is it in your role?** At the moment of writing this, I am a husband, brother, father, psychologist, and citizen. But all our roles are subject to change. Change is the constant. This is an example of how we can get attached to our identity and suffer when circumstances change because of our attachment to our prior identity. For example, a person very attached to their role at work can feel lost after retirement.
- **Is it in your thoughts?** To some extent, what we think influences who we are, because our thoughts influence our actions. However, you can think of one thing in this moment and, later today, another thing. We change our minds all the time. We believe one thing, reconsider, think another, have an experience that influences our thoughts, and so on.
- **Is it in your actions?** Our actions also are not constant, and sometimes aren't even consistent. You make mistakes and learn. You can have a persistent pattern of action and can change your actions. If I was usually doing that, and now I am doing this, then who am I? If a "bad man" does a "good thing," who is he? If I like to think of myself as a "good guy," but now I am acting with ill will toward you, then who am I?
- **Is it in your role in your society or religion?** Our culture can condition certain aspects of our identity in a way that, at first glance, can seem fixed. However, our conditioning can change with other experiences and contact with different cultures through our relationships or travel.
- **Is your ego your body?** We could say I am this body. Here I am. However, our bodies are constantly changing, even at the cellular level. I do not have the same body I had forty years ago. Am I still me? I recall a story about a young monk and

his teacher walking along the road when bandits set on them and beat both unconscious. The young monk awoke first and ran over to his master. Shaking him, he said, "Master, Master, are you okay?" The older monk answered, "This body is badly broken, but I am fine. Thank you."

When we perceive ourselves as having permanent traits and accept the illusion of being constant, we hold on to our ego and become attached to it. When people say, "This is just who I am," by misunderstanding their true selves, they significantly limit their potential for change. Clinging to the notion that *this is who I am* can sometimes be an excuse for resisting changes in how you do things.

When we become attached to our ego, we become more and more resistant to change. However, everything changes. When we free the mind from a fixed idea about who we are, we're open to change and changing circumstances. By letting go of our ego, we can see things more clearly and decrease our suffering.

We can also become attached to positive notions we incorporate into our ego. For example, I might get attached to the idea of being a "nice guy." But if I am grumpy and mistreat you, then who am I? If I am attached to my ego and you call me out for my unacceptable behavior, I will probably respond defensively. Much of our defensiveness is in the service of protecting the ego. If I am not attached to my ego, it is easy to be mindful of my temporary, destructive behavior, own it, and make a correction.

### Measuring the Ego

There is a troubling aspect to measuring the ego, and that is the arbitrariness of the activity. To decide whether I'm a good self, I have to determine what dimensions I will consider. I might decide to evaluate how successful I am, how wealthy I am, how intelligent or athletic I am, or how kind I am. Am I a nice guy or a jerk? I guess any combination of those would be a good start. However, why did I decide on those dimensions? What about hundreds of others I might have considered? Let's agree that the selection of dimensions to measure is arbitrary and is likely to be conditioned by family, culture, or circumstance.

Now, for any one dimension, I must decide on an *anchor point.* An anchor point is a cutoff where below falls short and above is a success. I might choose wealth as a dimension. As a psychologist, I make a good living compared to the general population. However, compared to a billionaire, I hardly have anything and am inadequate in the wealth-producing department. If I decide on athleticism as the dimension, I could think I am in good condition compared to other people my age. However, compared to a strong twenty-something, maybe not so much. I like to think of myself as kind, perhaps more than average. But I probably fall far short compared to someone like Mother Teresa. You can see that the choice of an acceptable anchor point is also arbitrary.

If we notice that these dimensions of self are arbitrary, and the anchor point selection is also arbitrary, it is wise to reconsider this whole measuring business. The more I measure, the more I keep getting caught in the pursuit of fixing this ego, this static sense of who I am when chasing an illusion. Everything moves, even if I do pin it down and settle on some dimensions and anchor points. Maybe I'm okay with my "self" today, but then I compare myself to another person, and suddenly I am no longer okay.

Perhaps if I select suitable dimensions and measure objectively with realistic anchor points, I can cultivate a positive sense of self with no problems. To some extent, this is true. However, this is a form of curing low self-esteem with high self-esteem. High self-esteem can present its own problems, usually derived from attachment to this new ideal view of myself. (Actually, we can also become attached to the idea of low self-worth.) The fundamental problem is that I am trying to measure something as if it is a static, tangible thing. Our ego is full of illusion, changing as conditions change.

We can notice that attaching experiences to the ego, viewing ourselves as having permanent, unchanging characteristics, and then trying to measure this ego, is filled with problems leading to suffering. When we do this, we experience things more and more in a "self-conscious" way, which inhibits us from being our best. We seem to be more effective, have more fun, and be more at peace when we are unselfconscious. The more we focus on the ego, the more we act in ways that serve and preserve it, which almost always leads to suffering.

So, if becoming preoccupied with the ego and *Who am I?* is not useful, what do we do instead?

### Measuring Actions

A frame to consider is "actions." The ego often feels like a heavy statue that we lug around. A lighter and more fluid way to be, is to focus on our immediate situation and our actions in that situation. By focusing on actions, you can be more attuned to whether your actions result in suffering. If so, you can adjust your actions. If not, you can continue as you were.

We have now identified two ways we can focus on things. One way is to focus on our ego. This can lead to a chain of consequences: I become preoccupied with the question *Who am I?* → I am unable to resist the urge to measure this ego to determine if it is adequate. → I become preoccupied with how other people measure my ego. → I become more and more attached to the ideas associated with my ego and act in ways that support it. → I suffer.

A second way of viewing things is to focus on our actions. In this case, I replace the question *Who am I?* with the question *What am I doing?* I am then mindful of my situation and my actions within this situation. The only thing I measure is how things are going. If they are going well (i.e., no suffering for me or others) then I proceed. If things aren't going well (someone is suffering) then I adjust my actions to align better with the situation. This view is lighter, and hence it's easier to adjust along the way. Lugging that ego statue around is exhausting and makes it hard to change course.

## Overcoming the Ego: No Longer Self-Conscious

If I am not attached to a notion about who I am, I am more able to align with circumstances as they change, and if I discover I'm not aligned, to adjust. In short, the "cure" for low self-esteem is not high self-esteem, but rather learning to view experiences without framing them as a reflection of self. We tend to feel better when we get out of the self-business.

One could argue that the root of much suffering is the egocentricity of identifying with a "me" as an unchanging separate self apart from things. When I get attached to this static self, I am always concerned about *serving the ego*. I become more preoccupied with what *I* want and how *I* think things should be. I get angry when other people or circumstances don't meet *my* expectations. I focus more and more on *me and mine*. Notice how we often use the possessive in our normal expressions. This is *my* child. This is *my* project. This is *my* house.

I hesitate to be the bearer of bad news, but the universe does not care who you are. It does not care who you think you are. But it seems to care about what you do.

When we understand the illusion of the ego, we notice the enormous amount of energy that goes into our preoccupations with it. Our thoughts tell a story about our experiences, with our ego as the main character. Every experience then becomes some reflection of who we are. When we let go of this notion, it all becomes lighter and easier to adjust. Think of times when you are the most at peace, the most effective, and experiencing the most joy. During these times, you were probably unselfconscious. When we are self-conscious and busily measuring ourselves, it impedes our ability to experience peace, joy, and effectiveness.

Sometimes we might think: *I would like to be a more confident person.* At first, this would seem like a worthwhile goal. It is arguably better to be a confident person than not. However, there is a subtle problem when we think about confidence this way. When I say I would like to be a confident *person*, I am framing it as though it is a permanent trait attached to my identity. We could view "being confident" as having an ongoing positive narrative in my head about my abilities. But I must be careful, because positive thoughts are only thoughts, and a narrative with myself as the chief topic is solely the churning of the ego. So how do we think about confidence without injecting an ego into the process?

One way is to think of confidence as "remembered mastery." If I think back on an experience where I handled a situation with success, I will feel confident when I consider doing that thing again and, to some extent, similar things. I regularly practice jiujitsu with people who are skilled and younger than me. I have a feeling of confidence at the thought of practicing with them because I have successfully done it so many times over the years. However, I have no experience in repairing a car engine, and so I would have no confidence in tearing down and rebuilding an engine. Confidence is not a static trait. It is a transient feeling related to remembered mastery as applied to new experiences that are similar to the ones in which we have experienced success. This differs from positive self-talk that is not necessarily grounded in any lived experience.

I might likewise want to be a "happy person." But again, this framing results in the same problem. I am striving to be a permanent ego that has the quality of "happy." I think, *If I can take this ego statue, scrape off all the mud, and shine it up, then it will shine forever.* Happiness results from conditions that are always changing. The more I strive for the permanent state of being a "happy person," the more I am disappointed. I may then even incorporate this disappointment into my ego, leading to the thought, *I am so disappointed in myself. What is wrong with me that I cannot be a permanently happy person? I suck.* This can relate to the problem of *toxic positivity*, which we will touch on in the next chapter.

I might strive for other ego expectations, such as being a successful businessperson or a successful parent. Again, the problem is seeking the permanent state. When we think this way, we often focus on the destination rather than the process. *I will be successful when I open my business. I will be a successful parent when my kid does X.* The seductive aspect to looking at things this way is expecting that when I arrive at the destination, all will be well. But when the feeling of satisfaction inevitably fades, I am disappointed. I open up my business, which feels successful at first, but then come the daily struggles. I feel like a successful parent when my child wins the award; then they become a teenager with testy, ever-changing moods, and I wonder where I went wrong.

It is not life changing that is the problem. It is our mind clinging that is the problem. It is essential to recognize when we are actually living our real life, and when we are caught up in the stories in our head. A man once said to the Buddha: "I want happiness." The Buddha said, "First remove 'I,' that's Ego, then remove 'want,' that's Desire. See, now you are left with only Happiness."

## Understanding Bounded vs. Unbounded

Some things are unbounded. Other things are bounded. This is reality. Compassion is unbounded, while our time, resources, energy, and influence are bounded.

Sometimes we face a situation where someone we care about is struggling. We recognize their suffering and feel deep compassion for their situation. Old souls and empaths experience this often. If we do not acknowledge what is bounded, our caring may take us to a place of suffering for both parties. It is essential to realize that we have limited energy and sometimes need to rest. We don't have unlimited resources to correct every deficit. I may discern a path for the person to move away from suffering, but I might be limited in my ability to influence the other person to see these possibilities.

When we have deep compassion for others, it is essential to remember that our compassion is incomplete if it does not include ourselves. If we keep serving the needs of others to the point where we ignore our own (e.g., our need for sleep or rest), eventually, things break down. Compassionate people can often get overwhelmed by the needs of those around them. Attending to their own needs is an afterthought. There is a story about a wise man being asked about the best way to see after the well-being of another. The answer was to "first see after your own." This was not an argument for selfishness, but an understanding that if you do not see after your well-being, eventually, you cannot see after the well-being of others. At the very least, you will not bring your best self.

Some people struggle with this problem of compassion by thinking they need to dial back their level of compassion. "I care too much; I need to be more hard-hearted." They may try this approach, but find it rarely works because it goes against their natural tendency to be compassionate. The solution is not to be less compassionate, but to be sure that you include yourself under that umbrella of compassion. I can feel deeply for another's suffering. My compassion for them, and all others, can be unbounded. But my time, energy, resources, and influence are bounded.

My passions and interests can also be unbounded. But again, my time, energy, and resources are bounded. Have you ever been in a public library and deeply considered how many books there are? You could stay nearly every day at the library reading and still only manage to read some of the books. This is the nature of things. We make choices. Every choice involves a loss. We create suffering when we try to "game the system" and avoid this reality by trying to find a choice that does not involve a loss.

## Understanding Boundaries

Part of Right Understanding, seeing things as they are, is understanding the concept of boundaries. There are entire books devoted to this one topic (e.g., Tawwab, 2021), and a full exploration of it is beyond the scope of this book. However, here is the gist: The psychological concept of boundaries refers to the limits we set in our relationships with others, both emotionally and physically.

There are different types of boundaries. *Physical boundaries* pertain to our bodies and personal space, including physical touch and personal property. *Emotional boundaries* pertain to our feelings and inner experiences. They include things like the level of intimacy we are comfortable with in relationships and which emotions we will share with others. *Mental boundaries* pertain to our thoughts, beliefs, and values and include how much influence we allow others to have over our decision-making.

Healthy boundaries are essential for maintaining healthy relationships and a sense of well-being. They allow us to control our lives and make the best choices. Having poor boundaries can lead to feeling overwhelmed, resentful, or taken advantage of. It can also lead to feelings of low self-esteem and self-worth.

Boundaries can be flexible and change over time, depending on the relationship, context, or personal growth. Establishing and maintaining healthy boundaries takes self-awareness and the ability to communicate effectively. Having clarity in one's mind about boundaries is vital for emotional well-being and good relations with others. When we have poor awareness of interpersonal, emotional, psychological, or physical boundaries, this lack of clarity is almost always associated with stress and suffering. So, what exactly is a boundary?

A boundary is an understanding of where one thing stops and another starts. There is a boundary that separates my property from my neighbor's. It is an understanding that on this side of the line is my property, and on the other is my neighbor's property. There might be a barrier on the boundary, like a big, well-constructed fence or a flimsy fence that barely stands upright. However, the fence is not the same thing as the boundary. The boundary is simply the understanding of the separation between one thing and another.

When we have clarity about the boundary, we also have clarity about ownership. It would be strange if I were to go over to my neighbor's property and rearrange their lawn furniture without permission. It would be odd because it's not my lawn furniture. Likewise, it would be strange if my neighbor were to come uninvited and rummage through my garage. Why? Because it's not theirs. When boundaries are clear, interactions between people are more peaceful. This is true in relationships with family, friends, and neighbors. It is also valid on a larger scale between nations. Where boundaries are clear, there is a greater tendency toward peace. Where boundaries are unclear, there tends to be more conflict.

Psychological boundaries refer to the idea that *I am not you.* I have thoughts, feelings, and needs. You also have thoughts, feelings, and needs. They may not be the same. I have not had the same journey in life that you may have had. We may do things differently. I might not do things that way, but I am not you. Remember, with clarity of boundaries comes clarity of ownership. If I have fuzzy boundaries, I might say, "You make me mad. What are you going to do to fix that?"

In my mind, the other person is not only the cause of how I feel, but they also bear the responsibility for fixing how I feel. I intend to remain angry and emotionally helpless until someone takes ownership of this problem. Well, that someone is me. Other people are not responsible for how I feel or how I deal with my suffering.

I struggle a bit with the notion of "setting boundaries." I prefer the term *clarifying boundaries*. It seems more complicated when we frame the exercise as "setting" boundaries. It seems as though, through force of will, I must put something in place that wasn't there before. This sounds more like a "fence" or a limit. The boundary does not have to be "set"; it is already there. It only must be acknowledged and thought about clearly. I understand I may sometimes interact with someone who operates within fuzzy boundaries. Still, if I have clarity in my mind about boundaries, I can approach the situation skillfully.

Simply remembering *I am not you* is a good starting point. If you start with this simple understanding, clarity of ownership and limits seems to occur naturally.

Things I might say to clarify boundaries:

*"That is a very interesting view. I don't happen to share it. I look at things this way."*

*"I wouldn't do things that way, but I am not you. You decide what works best for you."*

If someone says to me, "You make me mad," I could reply, "I am sorry that you are struggling with feeling angry, but I don't have the power to make you mad. You seem to be mad because of the way you choose to look at things. Is there any way I could support you while you sort through your anger?"

If someone wants to meet with me at 7 p.m., I could respond, "I'm sorry. I don't make appointments after 4 p.m."

Having clarity of boundaries allows you to be up close to the suffering of another without becoming confused. Clear boundaries make practicing compassion and loving-kindness toward someone else's suffering much easier.

Occasionally, someone in our life may be struggling. We have compassion for them, but it is difficult to watch the chaos in their life. You might visualize the other person as on a roller coaster going up and down, left and right, and sometimes in a scary fashion.

Your most effective stance is to imagine yourself firmly on the ground, stable, grounded, and centered. You choose not to get on the roller coaster with the other person. These are useful thoughts to have: *I have compassion for you. I probably would not do things that way. But I have clarity in the understanding that* I am not you.

It can be difficult to cope with someone who does not have clarity of boundaries. They sometimes need help to accept that you may have a different view or wish to do something other than what they want you to do. We might reply to their request with "I can't" when we mean "I don't wish to." But "I can't" implies that we would if we could, and this may invite the other party to quibble with your reasons until you feel you must say yes. It is better to reply more in line with how you actually feel: "I'd prefer not to." *Why?* "No special reason." It is harder to argue with a preference than with an excuse.

## Understanding the Illusion of the Road Not Traveled

We all go through life making a series of choices. We face a fork in the road and must choose to go in this direction or that direction. We continue our journey, choosing one way or another over and over again. Some of these forks in the road are trivial, and some are major crossroads. We decide to go after this career instead of the other one. We choose to marry this person rather than another, or not to marry at all. We have children, or we don't.

Our capacity for vivid imagination can help us to imagine solutions to problems or to plan for things. Sometimes we use our imagination to consider how life might have been had we chosen another road. We often imagine that road unfolding in a much better way than the road we chose. This vision of the road not traveled can be very detailed and often meets all our essential needs. The more we focus on this road, the more we grieve that rejected choice where everything worked out great.

The problem is that road only exists in our imagination. We are grieving the loss of something that never existed. *We have only one path.* It unfolds as a cumulative result of all the choices we have made along the way. We don't know the consequences of other choices, because those paths do not exist. We imagine everything would have turned out great, but we can never know in truth.

The illusion of the road not traveled often leads to grief related to losing that imagined path. It can also fuel a sense of regret. *I regret my choice, because I now experience the outcome of that choice.* We often use regret as a stick to beat ourselves with whenever we revisit the choice. Regrets are a heavy load that weighs us down as we move along the path we have chosen. But regrets can be helpful if we transform them into an intention to realize or learn something from the regret, and to use that understanding to move forward and avoid making the same mistake again.

I don't think that people intentionally make bad choices. *Hmm . . . Door #3 is full of suffering and will turn out badly . . . yeah, I think I'll pick that one.* Nobody does that. In the light of all our competing needs and considerations, Door #3 seemed like the best choice. Maybe we could not perceive at the time that Door #4 might have been a better choice, or maybe we couldn't perceive Door #4 at all.

When evaluating our prior selves, we often beat them up with some form of *What were you thinking?! Door #3! Really! What an idiot.* It may seem well-deserved, but it conveys a profound unfairness toward your prior self, who did not have the knowledge that your current self possesses. Your current self knows how the road unfolded. Your current self asks your prior self: "Couldn't you see that coming?" Prior self could respond, "Well, no. I couldn't."

## Understanding Destiny vs. Tendency

What if someone's parents and all four of their grandparents were alcoholics? Doesn't this mean they will be an alcoholic as well? Maybe someone comes from a long line of chaotic families ending with my crazy parents and siblings. Should they even bother getting married or having children?

There can be factors beyond our control that create conditions that make cultivating well-being more difficult. Genetic influences might make me more prone to alcoholism, depression, anxiety, or other major mental illnesses. My living situation may be a result of cumulative choices made by my ancestors, grandparents, and parents. Some would say I am destined to be alcoholic, or chaotic, or poor. It is unwise to pretend these factors do not encumber me to some degree.

However, it is essential to remember that there is a difference between destiny and tendency. You are not destined to become an alcoholic solely because your parents, grandparents, and earlier forebears were alcoholics. Being destined means there is no choice; it is your fate. Genetic and familial factors may influence you toward alcoholism. However, knowing this, you may decide to make choices that lead you in another direction.

## Understanding Overconfidence in What We Know to Be True

As human beings, we are inclined to perceive everything from the perspective of *How I see it is how it is*. We all are more confident in our perceptions than we should be. One study found that respondents who answered more factual questions correctly were more likely to agree with the scientific consensus about each topic. Those who answered many objective questions incorrectly but thought they understood specific topics well were more likely to disagree with the scientific consensus. For example, many who said that they would "definitely not get the vaccine" incorrectly answered questions about how viruses spread and how vaccines work, but then said they thought they had a "thorough understanding" of how a COVID-19 vaccine would work (Light, 2022).

"For many years, well-intentioned people thought that the way to bring people more in line with scientific consensus was to teach them the knowledge they lacked," the author of the study says. "Unfortunately, our research suggests that there may be a problem of overconfidence getting in the way of learning. . . . If people think they know a lot, they have minimal motivation to learn more" (Light, 2022). You might think that the cure for misinformation is accurate information. Unfortunately, research has shown that this is not the case.

Public attitudes that oppose scientific consensus can be disastrous when this dynamic is related to issues such as the rejection of vaccines and resistance to climate change mitigation policies. Five studies examining the interrelationships between opposition to expert consensus across seven critical issues that enjoy substantial scientific consensus, as well as attitudes toward COVID-19 vaccines and mitigation measures like mask-wearing and social distancing, found that those with the highest levels of opposition had the lowest levels of objective knowledge but the highest levels of subjective knowledge.

Research on overconfidence in beliefs is another area that argues for us to approach our views with humility, because of the relationship between overconfidence and mental health. We need to be reminded that *where there is perception, there can be deception.* Overconfidence in one's view is often associated with a mental rigidity that causes suffering. If I am overconfident in my views, I will be argumentative and judgmental. I will think I know better than anyone what is best. This rigidity not only leads to conflict with others, but also to stress, irritability, and anxiety.

It is perhaps counter-intuitive, but there is a sense of empowerment and true confidence that comes from saying, "I don't know." For example, I might say, "I know little about mRNA technology; that's outside my field." "I don't know, I have little experience with that." "I don't know what is best for you, because I'm not you." We live in a modern, complex world with many moving parts we don't fully understand (or at all). It is best to be humble and accept that. Being able to type keywords into a Google search box does not make me an expert. It makes me overconfident.

## Sometimes There Is No Understanding

There are good arguments for developing Right Understanding. If we take the time to focus on things with a clear mind, we understand how the world seems to work and can see things as they are. However, a great deal of life is filled with ambiguity and paradox. Our nature is to try to understand. We want answers, explanations, and understanding. An essential part of understanding is accepting that life is full of mysteries and that we don't always have an explanation for every question. There are some things that are hard to understand because words don't capture them well.

We often like to think that things happen for a reason. But sometimes things just happen. Usually, there is a complex matrix of reasons. Life, at times, makes little sense. We don't always have access to or understand all the factors at play. This is why we can be at a loss to explain another person's actions. We may not know all that they have experienced on their journey. It is important to be okay with not trying to explain everything that happens, and instead to embrace the ambiguities and paradoxes of life.

A Zen koan is a story, dialogue, question, or statement intended to provoke doubt and test a student's progress in Zen practice. The meaning of a koan is not meant to be understood intellectually, but to be realized through meditation and direct insight. Koans often have no logical or literal meaning and should challenge one's understanding of reality and consciousness.

Zen koans are often used to point to the limitations of our ordinary understanding and language, and to challenge our assumptions about reality and consciousness. By pushing beyond our usual ways of thinking, we can gain a deeper insight into the nature of things. Zen koans can be seen as a reminder that there are aspects of existence beyond our ordinary understanding, and that can only be experienced or realized through direct insight or spiritual realization.Top of Form

## The Path Forward . . .

Right Understanding is seeing things as they are and accepting the undeniable reality. Like the cherry blossoms, everything, both good and bad, is subject to change, so there's no sense in clinging. To see things as they are is to see how our minds cycle between wanting things to make us happy and not wanting things that make us uncomfortable. Our minds can also get caught in stubbornly refusing to accept things as they are and perpetually operating from willful ignorance. We explored our limitations as human beings because of perception and why it is important to practice humility about our subjective points of view. Central to understanding how things are is having a good understanding of ourselves and the differences between our ego and our actions. While Right Understanding is critical and there are a lot of important things to understand, sometimes things remain that we just don't understand.

Take a moment to reflect on Right Understanding. Consider taking some notes about whatever concept resonated with you. Is there a new understanding you could apply to your life now? Was there a concept you had never thought of before? How does thinking of it now change things for you?

In the next chapter, we will explore how our perspective is tied to how we think. We will explore many examples of how Right Understanding is reflected in clear thinking and a peaceful mind. We will also explore the many ways in which distorting how things are leads to distorted thoughts and consequent suffering.

*Calculate what man knows, and it cannot compare
to what he does not know.*
*-Chuang Tzu*

# 4

# RIGHT THOUGHT

*Your worst enemy cannot harm you*
*as much as your own thoughts, unguarded.*
*–Buddha*

# Buddhism and Right Thought

Right Thought follows directly from Right Understanding because our thoughts and intentions arise from our perception of reality. If you see reality as it is, you'll have no problems. But seeing reality through a haze of distorted perceptions, judgments, and concepts will lead to distorted thinking. So Right Thought is about investigating your thoughts and intentions to see if they align with reality—or not.

According to the Buddha, our thoughts are powerful; they determine our mental states, such as happy or sad, and then influence our actions. With Right Thought, you avoid the vicious cycle of craving and desire and the three "poisons" of desire, aversion, and ignorance. The more we keep our thoughts consistent with Right Understanding (seeing things as they are, not being deceived by perception, following the Middle Way), the more we plant the seeds of happiness and ethical conduct. By trying our best to keep our thoughts consistent with Right Understanding, we work at avoiding distorted thinking, we practice thoughts of compassion instead of anger or resentment, we avoid doing things in the service of the ego and instead are alert to reducing suffering in ourselves and others.

When practicing Right Thought, we must understand the duality of our human nature. We are capable of loving-kindness, but also anger and aggression. We can be peaceful and confident, but also fearful or jealous. Part of practicing is not pretending we are perpetually good at all times and don't have a darker nature, but rather openly acknowledging this, allowing us to notice it is arising before it goes too far. We can then gently cultivate more useful thoughts. Denying negative thoughts makes us much more vulnerable to their effects.

Cultivating thoughts of compassion toward others benefits not only others but also our own well-being. If I nurture thoughts of goodwill, then I am more likely to be aligned with Right Understanding. If I nurture thoughts of anger, resentment, revenge, hate, labels, and judgments, then I suffer from distorted thinking.

As we examine our thoughts, we can consider things like *Are these thoughts benefiting me and others? Are these thoughts coming from a place of fear or desire, or from a place of kindness? Are my thoughts serving my well-being or my ego?* Sometimes our thoughts imagine the future and our plans about how the road is supposed to unfold, or perhaps our fears about how it might unfold.

## Thoughts vs. Emotions

What is the difference between a thought and an emotion? Feelings and thoughts are distinct phenomena, but are also interrelated.

A *feeling* is a subjective experience that arises from within the body and can be characterized as a sense of pleasure, pain, tension, relaxation, excitement, calmness, and so on. Feelings are often accompanied by bodily sensations, such as changes in heart rate, breathing, muscle tension, and facial expressions. They are more immediate than thoughts.

A *thought* is a mental process that involves conscious awareness and can be characterized as an idea, belief, perception, opinion, memory, imagination, or reasoning. We often express thoughts in language that can be communicated to others. They are less immediate than feelings.

While feelings and thoughts are different phenomena, they are interconnected. Our thoughts can influence our feelings, and our feelings can influence our thoughts. For example, if we have negative thoughts about ourselves or others, it may lead to our experiencing negative feelings such as sadness, anxiety, or anger. Conversely, if we have positive feelings about a situation, we may feel pleasure or happiness.

Not all feelings result from thoughts. Some feelings can arise from sensory or physical experiences, such as feeling pain when we stub our toe or feeling pleasure when we eat our favorite food. I might have an anxious feeling from drinking too much coffee. These types of feelings are often more immediate and reflexive than those that are influenced by cognitive processes.

However, many feelings are indeed influenced by our thoughts and beliefs. For example, if we have a thought that something is dangerous, it can trigger a feeling of fear or anxiety. Similarly, if we have a thought that something is enjoyable, it can trigger a feeling of pleasure or happiness.

Our thoughts and beliefs can shape our emotional responses to events and situations, and they can also influence how we interpret and respond to those events and situations. In a Buddhist framework, Right Thoughts are those that promote a mental state of well-being as opposed to suffering. What are the "right" thoughts that cultivate a peaceful mind? Which thoughts are the right key to open the door to a space filled with well-being?

## Practicing Compassion

Compassion is a feeling of deep sympathy and empathy for someone who is experiencing pain, suffering, or hardship. It involves the desire to ease the suffering and to show kindness, understanding, and support. Compassion often involves a willingness to connect with others and to feel their pain as if it were one's own, leading to actions that aim to improve the situation of the person or group in need. Many cultures and religions throughout history have recognized compassion as a fundamental aspect of human nature.

Compassion can be both a feeling and a behavior. At its core, compassion is a feeling of empathy and concern for others who are suffering. However, we can also express compassion through behavior. When we act with compassion, we show kindness, empathy, and understanding toward others. This may involve offering emotional support, providing practical help, or simply showing care and concern.

In a Buddhist framework, compassion can be seen as a virtuous cycle, in which the feeling of empathy and concern motivates behavior that reinforces and strengthens the feeling. When we act with compassion, we not only help others but also experience a sense of purpose, connection, and well-being ourselves.

The Chinese government held the Tibetan monk Lopon la captive in a prison camp for eighteen years. They forced him to renounce his religion and tortured him many times. When asked what he most feared while in the prison camp, he said, "My greatest fear is that I would lose my compassion for my captors."

The more we practice a mindset of compassion toward others, the more we are aware of the reality that everyone suffers. We can see all sorts of suffering in our close relationships, in our community, and all over the world. The more we practice compassion, the more we know it is unbounded. We can have compassion for ourselves, our loved ones, people we only know casually, people we don't know directly, and even difficult and disagreeable people. We can practice compassion for those close to us and those on the other side of the world.

## Metta: The Practice of Loving-Kindness

One way to practice compassionate thoughts instead of thoughts reflecting anger or ill will is with Metta practice. In Pali, the language of the Buddha's teaching, loving-kindness practice is called *metta*. We can practice it in various ways, but one straightforward way is with a simple exercise that is helpful for people struggling with anger or resentment or a troublesome person. Here is an example:

1. Sit comfortably with your eyes closed. Pay attention to your breath, and allow it to settle into a comfortable and steady rhythm.
2. *Self*: First, consider yourself. Inhale and think, *I breathe in, knowing that I suffer.* Exhale and think, *I breathe out a wish to find whatever I need to be happy and well.* Repeat this four times.
3. *Loved One*: Next, think of a loved one. As you inhale, think, *I breathe in, knowing that they suffer.* As you exhale, think *I breathe out a wish they find whatever they need to be happy and well.* Repeat four times.
4. *Acquaintance*: Next, think of an acquaintance, someone you don't know well (e.g., the secretary in the other department, the neighbor three blocks away, the person who bags your groceries). Once you have a sense of them, continue the pattern. As you inhale, think, *I breathe in, knowing that they suffer.* As you exhale, think, *I breathe out a wish they find whatever they need to be happy and well.* Repeat four times.
5. *Difficult Person*: You reserve the last cycle for someone you struggle with. It could be someone who has hurt you or who is frustrating you. Continue with the same pattern: As you inhale, think, *I breathe in, knowing they suffer.* As you exhale, think, *I breathe out a wish they find whatever they need to be happy and well.* Repeat four times.
6. Then start again with another cycle of self, loved one, acquaintance, and difficult person. Repeat for however long you are devoting to the practice session.

Wishing that the difficult person find whatever they need to be happy and well can be, well, difficult. You might think: *You don't understand. I hate this person. I want them to suffer for what they have done. I want them to eat a sh*t sandwich and die!* Some people can be hurtful, mean, abusive, troublesome, or contrary. Our reflex is to wish them to suffer because they are making us suffer. We think, *I'll love my friends and family, but I'll never forgive that person who hurt me deeply.* We then realize that half-measures don't work so well. This practice helps us to realize that as long as we hang on to the wish that someone suffer, this causes within us our own suffering.

As we work through this metta practice, we can gradually learn to let go of our anger and ill-will toward people in our life who have caused us harm (see also the section on forgiveness in chapter 6). We develop an awareness that everyone suffers. Even the difficult person suffers from being difficult. Some people do an outstanding job being aware of other people's suffering and attentive to their well-being, but not such a great job including themselves in their practice. If your compassion does not include yourself, it is incomplete.

# CBT and Right Thought

*"The problem is not the problem.*
*The problem is your attitude about the problem. Do you understand?"*
*– Jack Sparrow*

## Thoughts vs. Feelings

There are different ways we can consider feelings. We mentioned earlier that some feelings are generated from the midbrain area and are automatic, occurring without thought. If a bear suddenly jumps out at you, the startle reflex you experience doesn't require any thought process. It is automatic.

We also understand that many feelings can have a neuro-chemical aspect. Mental health disorders such as anxiety, depression, or bipolar disorder can have a tremendous impact on how we feel because of imbalances in neurotransmitters in the brain. Hormonal changes can induce feelings of irritability, sadness, and anxiety. We might feel anxious after having too much coffee or happy when using certain drugs.

Other feelings may result from thought. Our interpretation of a situation can lead to a series of thoughts, which become a narrative. This narrative is the engine behind how we feel. For example, I might think about an upcoming meeting at work, picture all the ways the meeting could go poorly, and then feel anxious. Feelings derived from our interpretations have a psychological origin as opposed to a phys-iological or neurochemical origin. For most of the remaining chapter, we will focus on feelings that result from thoughts—those with a psy-chological origin.

In the Buddhist framework, Right Thought is in alignment with Right Understanding. Essentially, we see reality without distortion, and our thoughts align with this clear understanding. A CBT framework has a very similar approach. In this framework, negative emotional states are thought to derive from distorted perceptions about events. As in Right Understanding, when we don't see things clearly, we suffer.

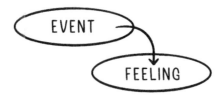

In casual conversation, we often say things like: "This happened, and it made me feel . . .," "The meeting is tomorrow, and it is making me anxious," or "He said X, and it made me mad." In casual conversation, most people understand what you mean when you say these things. There is some connection between this thing that happened or might happen and how you feel. What we imply in stating things this way is that the relationship between the event and the feeling is a direct causal line. The event *made me* feel.

When we view our emotional experience in this fashion, it severely limits us in being able to change how we feel. If the event is *making* me feel, what am I to do? I have no choice in the matter. This frame leads to relying on two strategies to deal with the feeling. The first is to find a distraction. If I find something to focus on that is engaging enough so I won't think about what is bothering me, I will get some relief. This strategy works to an extent. The problem is that the activity I am concentrating on must have greater engagement energy than the energy of the issue distressing me. The second strategy is to wait for the issue to run out of energy. This also works sometimes. Wait long enough, and this too shall pass. However, sometimes it can take a long time for the energy to dissipate, and I might spend days suffering unnecessarily.

The basic CBT model would suggest that a simple *event-causes-feeling model* differs from how our feelings operate. There is a step between the event and the resulting feeling. This step is perception. A more accurate model of how our feelings work is:

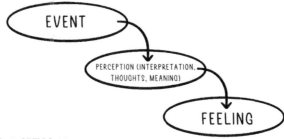

*Figure 4: Basic CBT Model*

In this model, events don't *make us* feel in a direct causal line. Events happen. After they happen, we assign meaning to them, interpret them, and have thoughts about them. This step of perception then generates one or more emotions.

Now to expand the model a bit:

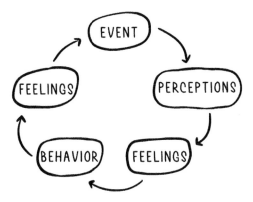

*Figure 5: Expanded CBT Model*

Events happen, and we assign meaning to them. This meaning affects how we feel (and therefore these feelings are of a psychological, as opposed to neurochemical or physiological, nature), how we feel affects our behavior, and how we behave affects our feelings. Our behavior and feelings may then create subsequent events.

Many studies have found this to be a robust model. The natural extension of this model is then to ask: What about when people have negative emotions such as anxiety, anger, or depression? Are there any perceptual patterns that seem to accompany these negative mood states? The answer is yes. These perceptual patterns are called *cognitive distortions.*

## Cognitive Distortions

Cognition is a fancy way of saying a thought. A cognitive distortion is a thought that seems out of alignment with reality. Because of this lack of alignment, we cannot see things clearly. This lack of alignment with how things are appears to routinely generate distress. In this sense, in the Buddhist framework, the thoughts are out of alignment with Right Understanding. These distortions are simply ways in which our mind convinces us of something that is not true.

These inaccurate thoughts are usually used to reinforce negative thinking or emotions. The thoughts seem rational and accurate, but they only generate suffering. It is hard to stay in accord with Right Understanding if our thoughts constantly distort our perception, making it very difficult to see things as they are.

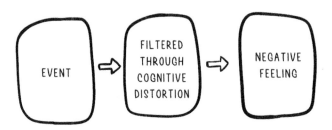

Below are some common cognitive distortions (Burns, 1980). Nobody does all these all the time. We may find that a handful are ones we do regularly and are a significant cause of our suffering. Each of the cognitive distortions has a reason for being "distorted." Each also has specific ways it can be *reframed*. In reframing, we work at recognizing the lie in the distortion and correcting it.

I encourage learning the name of each cognitive distortion and its corresponding definition. This is not to prepare for some test (although life is a test of sorts . . . but I digress). Rather, sometimes we only have a vague sense that we aren't thinking in a helpful way, but no clear direction for how to correct it. It is helpful to be more precise in our investigation. What exactly are you thinking right now? Does your negative emotion give any clue which specific cognitive distortion might be affecting your perception? When we can name something, it is easier to perceive it. Here are the most common cognitive distortions:

1. **All-Or-Nothing Thinking.** You see things as black and white. If your performance falls short of perfection, you see yourself as a total failure. Someone either loves you or they don't. They either trust you entirely or not at all. The distortion arises from forcing things that occur on a continuum into "either/or" categories— there is no middle ground, no shades of gray. All-or-nothing thinking doesn't allow for the complexity of most people and situations.
   * *Reframe:* Avoid categorical words and use words that convey degree. For example, instead of "trust or not," show the degree of trust and in which areas. Use words and phrases that reflect the

grey areas. All-or-nothing thinking is a distortion because most things we deal with are not categorical or binary. Avoiding the distortions accompanying extreme frames is part of practicing the Middle Way. With practice, it gets easier to identify all-or-nothing language and to phrase things as a matter of degree.

2. **Mind Reading.** You arbitrarily conclude that someone is reacting negatively to you, without checking whether that conclusion is true. We imagine what someone is thinking, feeling, or intending, and then treat what we imagine as fact. We put thoughts into the other person's mind, and then react to them as though it's a fact. The distortion is that we cannot read minds. We guess, and we are often wrong.

• *Reframe*: Try to get comfortable with the phrase "don't know." Instead of speculating what someone is thinking, feeling, or intending—replace this with "don't know." We can't read minds, so believing that we can is out of sync with reality. "Why is he acting that way?" Answer: "Don't know." Don't know is most in alignment with reality. If I start with, "don't know," I can ask the other person their thoughts, feelings, or intentions, and then I can know.

Occasionally practice making up stories. Why was that person rude? Hmmm, they may be a bad person who is rude to everyone. Maybe they have a headache or don't feel well. Perhaps Grandma is in the hospital, and they are preoccupied. Maybe they are mind reading and putting thoughts into *my* head. When you make up stories, it reminds you that people exist in a larger context. The more you "make up" stories, the more you can recognize that is precisely what mind reading is. One story is as good as another.

3. **The Fortune Teller Error.** You imagine how the road is going to unfold. You expect things will turn out badly, and you feel convinced that your prediction is already true. The distortion is that we don't know the future with any certainty. One problem of fortune telling is that it can lead to a self-fulling prophecy. For example, you convince yourself that a colleague at work is mad at you. Because of this belief, you might be stilted or terse in your interactions with the colleague. The colleague eventually becomes annoyed and says so. You then congratulate yourself on how perceptive you are, completely unaware of how your actions brought on the thing you were predicting.

• *Reframe:* The correction of this cognitive distortion is similar to that for mind reading. Just as you *cannot read minds*, you *cannot predict the future*. You know your past; you don't know how the road ahead will unfold. Because the future is unknown, you are most aligned with reality when you get comfortable with "don't know."

How's that meeting going to go? Don't know. What's going to happen when you confront your friend? Don't know. Often people will say, "You don't understand. When I don't know is when I am the most anxious." It is essential to realize is that it is not the *fact* that something is unknown that makes you anxious. You're anxious because you have a tendency as a human being to want to fill in the blank with a story. Most of the time, you choose a story that makes you anxious. A blank slate is not as scary as an elaborate story.

4. **Magnification (Catastrophizing) or Minimization:** You exaggerate the importance of things (such as your goof-up or someone else's achievement). Or you inappropriately shrink things until they appear tiny (your desirable qualities or the other person's imperfections). This is also called the "binocular trick." Some examples of catastrophizing:

   *"If I fail this test, I will never pass school and be a total failure in life."*
   *"If I don't recover quickly from this procedure, I will never get better and be disabled my entire life."*
   *"If my partner leaves me, I will find no one else, and I will never be happy again."*

   Minimizing is when we downplay the significance of something. For example, Mary's friend was yet another person to tell her she thought Mary was drinking too much and putting herself in danger. Mary dismissed her concerns by saying, "You're like everyone else. You worry too much," and she thought, *I don't know what they're all so worried about.*

   • *Reframe.* When we view things in isolation and without context, they can seem psychologically "large" or "small" in a distorted way. One way to challenge this distortion is to add events for comparison. Rate the event on an "awful" index from 0 to 100. Then, to provide perspective, add to the scale other events you have or experienced or could experience.

   Losing your job is tragic, like a ninety-five on the awful index. You might stay with this experience of the event as a ninety-five if you stay with the tunnel vision that can occur when you're stressed. The way to overcome the tunnel vision is to add other events. Ask yourself, *How does this compare to other times I have left a job? How would this compare to the loss of a loved one? Loss of my sight?* Put this new event in the context of similar events you've experienced or could experience.

5. **Emotional Reasoning:** You assume that your negative emotions reflect how things are. Emotional reasoning takes emotion as evidence of truth. Burns argues that this is backward, because your feelings reflect [are a product of] your thoughts and beliefs and are therefore invalid. After all, if our thoughts are biased, then emotions experienced as a result of those thoughts don't correspond to the world as it is. Examples of emotional reasoning include feeling hopeless and concluding that a problem is impossible to solve, or feeling angry and concluding that another person is acting badly. You assume that your unhealthy emotions reflect how things are: I feel it; therefore, it must be true.

   • *Reframe:* What evidence do you have that shows reality is inconsistent with your emotion? What other factors might account for the emotion? Could internal factors account for it? Ask yourself, *Am I anxious because I had too much coffee?*

6. **Should Statements:** We have a list of ironclad rules about how others and we should behave. People who break the rules make us angry, and we feel guilty when we violate these rules. You try to motivate yourself with should, as if you had to be whipped and punished before you could be expected to do anything. "Musts" and "oughts" are also offenders. The emotional consequence is guilt. When you direct should-statements toward others, you feel anger, frustration, and resentment. I should not have spent so much money. I must always exceed expectations. They shouldn't be doing that.

   • *Reframe:* Try saying what you want to say but without using the word "should" or any of its synonyms. For example, you might say, "I should have studied harder." Perhaps you should have, but what do you want to do about that now, if anything? Or you might say, "They shouldn't be acting that way." Maybe they shouldn't. But they are. Is there anything to be done? There is no value added by the should statement; it only makes you annoyed or regretful. Better to just have the problem without the extra layer of annoyance.

7. **Labeling and Mislabeling:** This is an extreme form of over-generalization. We generalize one or two qualities into a negative global judgment. Instead of describing an error in a specific

situation, a person will attach an unhealthy label to themselves. For example, when they fail at a specific task, they may say, "I'm a loser." When someone else's behavior rubs a person the wrong way, they may attach an unhealthy label to them, such as "He's a real jerk." Mislabeling involves describing an event with language that is highly colored and emotionally loaded. For example, instead of saying someone drops her children off at daycare every day, someone mislabeling might say that "she abandons her children to strangers."

- *Reframe:* Ask yourself what the label you are using exactly means. We often use a word with a negative connotation without thinking about the actual definition. Labeling is a distortion because it takes a person or situation that is fluid and changing and describes it as something permanent or static. Remember the Buddhist concept of impermanence. What does it mean to define ourselves as "inferior," "a loser," "a fool," or "abnormal?" If you examine these and other global labels, you will probably discover that they represent specific behaviors or an identifiable behavior pattern rather than the whole person. To address mislabeling trying to notice the judgmental tone. Is the thought coming from a neutral place or an angry one?

8. **Personalization:** You see yourself as the cause of an adverse event that you were not primarily responsible for. You imagine you are the sole reason other people do what they do. You also compare yourself to others, trying to determine who is more intelligent, better looking, and so forth. For example, "We were late to the dinner party and caused the hostess to overcook the meal. This wouldn't have happened if I had only pushed my husband to leave on time."

- *Reframe:* We typically learn this personalization distortion when we are raised in an environment where people often project blame onto others. For example, caregivers may have said, "You make me mad." If you receive a lot of projected blame, you can develop a reflex where you feel as if you are the cause for another person's feelings. What other factors might cause others to do what they do besides you being the root cause? We often forget that other people live a complex life with many moving parts, just as we do. They have unique journeys with uncountable influences that might affect how they respond to any situation.

9. **Control Fallacies:** If we feel externally controlled, we see ourselves as helpless and a victim of fate. For example,

"I can't help it if the quality of the work is poor. My boss demanded I work overtime on it." The fallacy of internal control has us assuming responsibility for the pain and happiness of everyone around us. For example, "Why aren't you happy? Is it because of something I did?"

- *Reframe*: You only have control from your fingertips back. If you try to control other people or situations to regulate how you feel, this will often lead to anger and frustration. You only have control over yourself. "Out there" is beyond your control. Reframing control as being directed only toward yourself does not mean you have to adopt a passive stance. You might respond passively, assessing that there is nothing to be done. Or you might respond actively but only control your actions. It is usually very calming to clarify control for ourselves. You can adopt this mantra: *There is nothing "out there" that I have control over. I only have control over how I respond to "out there."*

10. **Fallacy of Fairness:** We feel resentful because we know what is fair, but others won't agree. As our parents tell us, "Life isn't always fair." People who go through life measuring every situation, judging its "fairness," will often feel bad and negative as a consequence.
- *Reframe:* Try to view the situation without measuring its fairness. What, if anything, is to be done, regardless of whether the situation is fair? It might not be fair, but you may still have to deal with it in some fashion. Sometimes, there may be a mechanism for addressing a lack of fairness. Other times, things just happen. It is essential to understand that the universe is not keeping score, passing out misfortune in equal doses to everyone. Sometimes you can do everything right and still have a bad outcome.

11. **Blaming:** You blame other people for your pain, or take the other tack and blame yourself for every problem. For example, "Stop making me feel bad about myself." Nobody can "make" you feel any particular way—only you have control over your emotions and emotional reactions, because you control the meaning you choose to give what you are experiencing.
- *Reframe*: Try to avoid making other people the cause of how you feel. If you say things like "You make me mad," you are putting the root cause of your feelings in the other person. You can't control other people, but you can control how you react to other people. If you remind yourself that your emotional response arises from how you view the situation—i.e., your perspective, you have more control over your reaction.

12. **Fallacy of Change:** You expect other people to change to suit you if you pressure or cajole them enough. You need to change people because your hopes for happiness depend entirely on them changing. When you frame things this way, you put the control of your emotions onto external situations. This can set up a feeling of helplessness or frustration.

- *Reframe:* Trying to change others to change your feelings leads to feeling frustrated or helpless, because you are trying to control something that you have no control over. Instead of thinking, *I'll be happy just as soon as so-and-so changes,* ask yourself, *Why am I not happy even if they do not change?*

13. **Always Being Right:** You are continually on trial to prove your correct opinions and actions. Being wrong is unthinkable, and you will go to any length to show your rightness, even with loved ones. For example, "I don't care how bad arguing with me makes you feel. I will win this argument no matter what, because I'm right." Sometimes we fall into this distortion when we don't understand the difference between things that are subjective and things that are objective.

- *Reframe:* Ask yourself, *Do I want to be right or happy?* Sometimes we pursue being right at the expense of our happiness and that of those around us. Ask yourself what it means to you if you are right, but others can't accept that. Ask yourself whether you are applying "right and wrong" to something that is subjective or a matter of opinion. Is loving-kindness driving the conversation, or your ego?

*14. Heaven's Reward Fallacy*: Psychologist Aaron Beck described the heaven's reward fallacy as "expecting all sacrifice and self-denial to pay off as if someone were keeping score, and feeling disappointed and even bitter when the reward does not come." The irrational belief that the universe will somehow reward all your sacrifices may seem comforting. It can promise hope for positive consequences. But not all effort or hard work gets rewarded. Not all sacrifices will entitle you to a reward. And not all sacrifices will be redeemed by the universe. Heaven's reward might be a comforting thought, but it can lead to disappointment and judgments like "Life is too unfair."

In most cases, it is a reasonable belief that results depend on hard work and sacrifice. But an exaggerated version of that— your hard work will make you succeed *no matter what*—is the heaven's reward fallacy.

- *Reframe:* Ask yourself why you feel bitter if your sacrifice and self-denial are not "paying off." Are you angry at some cosmic scorekeeper? Are you doing things as an end in themselves or to get some "payoff?" Behaving in a kind manner seems to be a good way to be. However, if you act in a kind manner and you want to be appreciated or admired for it, the motivation behind your kindness is the problem, not the kindness itself. Sometimes you can do all the right things, *just with the wrong person.*

## Origins of Cognitive Distortions

Sometimes people ask, "Why do I have these cognitive distortions?" That's an excellent question. A common source of cognitive distortions is what we hear growing up. If you had a parent who was often critical, who overgeneralized or labeled you with mean names, you would likely develop thought patterns that mirrored this speech. The speech does not even have to be directed toward you. Suppose we grow up sitting around the dinner table and hearing conversation that reflects all-or-nothing thinking, mind reading, labeling, and other distortions. We can then internalize that thinking. Growing up, we develop our fundamental beliefs about relationships and how they work by observing relationships around us.

Cognitive distortions are also an outgrowth of not understanding reality clearly. Even the basic idea that our perceptions can be faulty and deceive us if not understood can lead to distorted thoughts. One common problem is being overly confident and unquestioning of one's perceptions. When I make this mistake, I think everything I view is objective. How I see things is directly how it is. Suppose this is my starting point about how reality works. In that case, my thought process will inevitably be highly rigid, out of alignment with reality, and as a result, a powerful engine for suffering.

## Tools for Correcting Cognitive Distortions

It is a good start to be aware of the notion of cognitive distortions and the impact they can have on our well-being. However, we need to do more than simply be aware of cognitive distortions. It is crucial to recognize them when they occur, and then to actively practice correcting the distortions. There are several ways to challenge and correct cognitive distortions. Here are a few examples.

## 3-Column Technique (Burns, 1980)

Recall the basic CBT model:

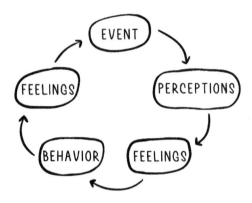

*Figure 6: Basic CBT Model*

The 3-column technique is a method of deconstructing upsetting events. One study found that simply labeling the emotion associated with an event, without the intention of changing the emotion at all, will cause some downregulation of the emotion. This effect was demonstrated in self-reported distress and brain activity in the brain's stress centers (Burklund, 2014). In addition, because our thoughts bounce around like ping-pong balls, especially when we are upset, writing makes it easier to see the threads that connect one thought to another. The end thought might be far away from where you started, but it may be the thought that is primarily driving your feelings.

Here are the steps in the 3-column technique:

1.  *Describe the upsetting event.* In your journal, describe an event that you are feeling reactive toward. Use objective terms with no layer of interpretation. For example, you might write, "My coworker said, 'Your presentation could have been better,'" as opposed to "A coworker said my presentation in the meeting was lame and it made me mad." Take the time to notice layers of interpretation and get used to simply stating what happened.
2.  *Record your negative feelings.* Identify the feelings you are having and describe them using specific language. For example, if you feel angry, is it a hurt kind of anger (perhaps resentment) or a frustrated kind of anger (perhaps irritability or exasperation)? This verbal labeling process begins to downregulate emotional reactivity.

3.  *Fill out the three columns.* Reproduce the three columns below in your journal and fill in each column.

| NEGATIVE THOUGHTS | DISTORTIONS | REPHRASE |
|---|---|---|
| WRITE THE THOUGHTS THAT MAKE YOU UPSET. | IDENTIFY ANY COGNITIVE DISTORTIONS IN THE THOUGHTS YOU WRITE DOWN. | SAY WHAT YOU WANT TO SAY BUT WITHOUT THE DISTORTION. |

A.  In the first column, write your thoughts in a stream-of-consciousness fashion. In other words, don't edit yourself or approach the task as if someone is reading over your shoulder. Just let the thoughts flow. You may be used to thinking at 110 miles per hour, but find you can only write at ten miles per hour. While this is frustrating, it is also a benefit. By slowing down in the writing, you will find your thoughts also slow down. You will then be more able to notice threads that connect your thoughts and see how these connections relate to how you feel. It is often good when upset about something to first slow down.
B.  Take a pause, and then read what you wrote. Now you are in observer mode. Observing your thoughts is a very different thing from experiencing your thoughts, and the powerful psychological shift that occurs cannot be overstated. In observer mode, you can more critically examine your thoughts. Are there any examples of cognitive distortions? If so, identify the specific cognitive distortion by name in this second column. Once you can identify the specific cognitive distortion by name, you can push back and reframe.
C.  In the third column, work on reframing your thoughts about the event. Say whatever you want to say, but try to say it without cognitive distortions. This last step is not "positive thinking" to replace "negative thinking." It is not an attempt to adopt a pollyannish outlook where everything is puppies and rainbows. It is not striving toward toxic positivity. Sometimes events are unfortunate. But is it a catastrophe? This step seeks to replace distorted thinking with thoughts that better aligned with reality.

It is common when beginning this process to emphasize changing the content of the thoughts from negative to positive in an attempt to have "better" thoughts. *Don't merely change the content. Change the filter.* For example, don't replace negative fortune-telling with positive fortune-telling. Avoid fortune-telling altogether. In the third column we can use the reframing techniques we discussed earlier.

### Arrow Technique

Sometimes the thoughts we can identify do not account for the depth of how we feel. There may be a more substantial core belief that the surface thought it is tapping into. Whenever the thoughts we are aware of don't seem to account for the depth of the emotion we are experiencing, this might be a good time to try the arrow technique.

With the arrow technique, you drill down and try to identify the thoughts that underlie the surface thoughts you are aware of.

1. Start by grabbing your journal and writing the initial automatic thought.
2. Next, operate as though that thought were true, and ask yourself what it would mean.
3. When you have your answer, ask yourself the same question again. If this second thought were true, what would that mean?
4. Repeat this line of questioning until you understand the core belief that resonates with the current situation.

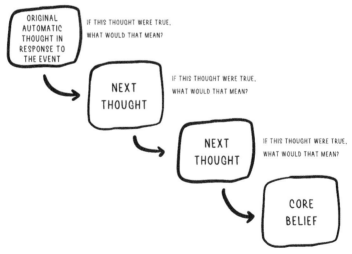

*Figure 7: Arrow Technique*

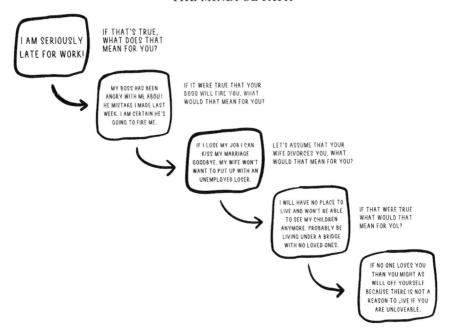

*Figure 8: Arrow Technique example*

In this example, the person can better understand their acute distress at simply being late for work, because the initial thoughts were tapping into the long-standing core belief of being unlovable. Over time, by making these connections, we can understand the roots of our core beliefs and correct them.

## Examine the Evidence

A thorough examination of an experience allows us to identify the basis for our distorted thoughts. Many times, we look for evidence that supports our thoughts. This can lead to what is called the confirmatory bias. Looking for evidence that does *not* support your thought is critical to correct this bias.

Here are some questions to help find evidence that does not support your thought from *Mind Over Mood* by Greenberger and Padesky (1995):

• Have I had any experiences showing that this thought is not always entirely true?
• If my best friend or someone I loved had this thought, what would I tell them?
• If my best friend or someone who loves me knew I was thinking this, what would they say? What evidence would they point out that

would suggest my thoughts were not one hundred percent true?
- When I am not feeling this way, do I think about this type of situation any differently? How?
- When I have felt this way in the past, what did I think that helped me to feel better?
- Have I been in this type of situation before? What happened? Is there anything different between this situation and the previous one? What have I learned from my previous experiences that could help me now?
- Are any small things contradicting my thoughts that I might discount as unimportant?
- If I look back on this situation five years from now, will I look at it differently? Will I focus on any different part of my experience?
- Are there any strengths or positives in me or the situation I am ignoring?
- Am I jumping to any conclusions not entirely justified by the evidence?
- Am I blaming myself for something I do not entirely control?

### Double Standard Method

An alternative to "self-talk" that is harsh and demeaning is to talk to ourselves in the same compassionate and caring way in which we would speak with a friend in a similar situation. Imagining ourselves talking to someone in a similar situation helps us to observe when we have one standard (usually rigid and harsh) that we hold ourselves to and another more forgiving one for others. It's hard to imagine telling a friend: "I can't believe you made a mistake. You are such an idiot. You know things are going to fall apart now. Everyone probably thinks you're an idiot." It would feel unkind to treat someone that way, but sometimes we talk to ourselves that way in our private thoughts. By the way, if you have a friend or anyone that speaks to you that way, carefully consider where the relationship fits into your journey.

### Thinking in Shades of Gray

Instead of thinking about our problem or predicament in an either-or-polarity, evaluate things on a scale of 0–100. When you did not fully realize a plan or goal, consider the experience a partial success on a scale of 0–100. If an event is adverse, score it on an "awful" scale of 0–100. Add other events on the scale to allow for calibration and perspective. For example, you might have been passed over for promotion and, in your despair, rate the awfulness of this experience as a ninety-five. How would you rate the loss of the job altogether? How about the loss of a loved one? How about other negative experiences you have had? Adding other events allows for a broader perspective of the experience. Usually, we magnify things when we lose the broader context.

## Survey Method

We sometimes need to seek the opinions of others regarding whether our thoughts and attitudes are realistic. If we say something to ourselves like *I'm sure everyone is thinking . . .*, we can survey by asking a handful of people if they do actually think that, and if so, what percentage do? If you believe your anxiety about an upcoming event is unwarranted, check with a few trusted friends or relatives to get their perspective.

## Cost-Benefit Analysis

Listing the advantages and disadvantages of feelings, thoughts, or behaviors is helpful. A cost-benefit analysis will help us find out what we gain from feeling bad, distorted thinking, and inappropriate behavior. I was angry and yelled at my partner. What do I get out of this behavior? How does this work for me? How does it work against me? Do I enjoy a short-term or immediate benefit but suffer a long-term cost?

## Correcting Beck's Cognitive Triad

Recall Beck's Cognitive Triad that he noticed was common to his patients with depression.

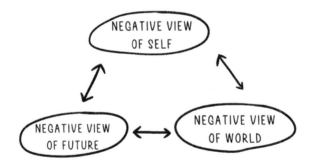

*Negative View of Self:* Practice resisting framing experiences in terms of self. Understand that the nature of the ego is an illusion of something permanent or static. View yourself as a verb instead of a noun. Ask yourself, *What am I doing, and how is that going?* versus *Who am I, and is that adequate or not?*

*Negative View of Future:* Practice becoming comfortable with uncertainty. Leave unknowns as unknowns instead of trying to fill in the blank. Let the future unfold as it will. Center your focus on the present.

*Negative View of the World:* Practice letting go of the wish to control things beyond the ends of your fingertips (i.e., everything out in the world). Remember that your compassion is boundless, but your time, energy, resources, and influence are bounded. As Gandhi said: "Be the change you want to see in the world."

## Toxic Positivity

When correcting distorted thinking, the effort is not directed toward turning negative thinking into positive thinking. Looking at things through a negatively distorted filter is certainly not helpful. It is also useless to look at things through a positively distorted filter.

*Toxic positivity* is when somebody pretends that everything is going well even when it is not. It is when they avoid all negative thoughts or feelings. "Just think positively!" "It could be worse." "You should look at the bright side!" "Don't worry, be happy."

Psychotherapist Whitney Goodman describes toxic positivity as the "unrelenting pressure to be happy and positive, no matter the circumstances" (Goodman, 2022). We may bring it onto ourselves by not allowing negative thoughts and feelings, but it's also something we can cause other people to experience. I relate toxic positivity to the Buddhist concept of aversion. Recall that aversion is negatively judging other people or our own emotions. *I hate it when I feel that way. I hate it when others feel that way.* Expressing toxic positivity to others may occur in the form of offering them a simple solution to a complicated problem we know nothing about, or not allowing people around you to appropriately express negative sentiments. Toxic positivity can happen around issues like infertility, parenthood, and especially mental health. Sometimes well-intentioned people might say to someone who is depressed something like: "Well, maybe if you learned to look on the bright side you wouldn't struggle with depression so much." Or they might say to a parent struggling with a difficult child: "Maybe if you taught them how to behave, there wouldn't be so many problems." Similarly with anxiety: "If only you didn't worry so much, you wouldn't be anxious." Having trouble with infertility? "Don't worry. You will have a child when it is God's will." (In other words, if you can't get pregnant, God hates you.)

Toxic positivity can be harmful because it causes us to suppress our emotions, which can worsen them. "They become more intense and can also lead to long-lasting health concerns in the future," Goodman says. Denying issues and trying to will them away with positive thinking can keep us stuck. This dynamic of shutting down negative emotions can occur in some families. If this was your dynamic while growing up, you might continue the practice as an adult.

If you're using toxic positivity against yourself, it is essential to remember that it is OK to experience negative emotions sometimes. In Buddhist thought, the Middle Way is a significant insight. We don't want to immerse ourselves in negative emotions, nor should we be averse to experiencing them when they are present.

## Cognitive Biases

Another group of thinking errors we often experience are *cognitive biases*. Cognitive biases are like cognitive distortions in that they distort our perceptions and make it hard to see things as they are. A cognitive distortion is more of a learned habit in thinking and is amenable to change. Cognitive biases are more related to ways we process information that are "hardwired" in our brains through evolution and that most anyone can be prone to. We evolved in a very complex world with lots of information to process. Having simple rules of thumb to help us navigate this world can provide an evolutionary advantage. It also protects our brain from cognitive overload. However, while rules of thumb can simplify matters, they can also lead to systematic biases. Here are a few examples.

### Confirmation Bias

When caught in *confirmation bias*, we start with our already drawn conclusion and then seek evidence that supports our view. This differs from starting off neutral and seeing how things shake out on all sides. When we are caught in this bias, we give more weight to things that support what we already believe and neglect or dismiss evidence that doesn't support our view.

Common characteristics of confirmation bias include an unwillingness to accept the validity of evidence that defies my previously held beliefs. For example, I place greater weight or emphasis on "facts" that appeal to my underlying assumptions, to the exclusion of contradictory evidence. I actively seek information that "proves" my point. I selectively and often incorrectly recall events, facts, or statistics.

Confirmation bias can make people more likely to dismiss information that challenges their views. A recent study of millions of Facebook users found that many preferred to get their news from a few sources they already agreed with (Schmidt, 2017). Even when people are exposed to contrary information, confirmation bias can cause them to reject it and, unfortunately, become even more confident that their beliefs are correct (Nickerson, 1998).

One famous experiment gave students evidence from two scientific studies—one that supported capital punishment and one that opposed it. The students disputed whichever study went against their pre-existing opinion and embraced their original position even more passionately.

Studies have shown that even clinicians can fall into this bias. When making a diagnosis, a physician may look for things are consistent with the diagnosis they suspect. This is called *confirmatory hypothesis testing*. They may fail to look for things that don't fit.

### Negativity Bias

The *negativity bias* is a cognitive bias that results in adverse events more significantly impacting our mental state than positive events. This bias causes our emotional response to negative events to feel magnified compared to similar positive events. This magnification effect is then linked to *loss aversion*, a cognitive tendency that describes why the pain of losing is psychologically twice as powerful as the pleasure of gaining.

Negativity bias appears to be a natural adaptive function developed during evolution. By continually being exposed to threats to survival, like predators thinking of lunch, our ancestors developed a negativity bias to survive (Vaish, 2008). We have significant brain resources devoted to noticing what needs to be corrected, what is out of place or not as it should be, and threats. Things that are in place, not threatening, just as they should be, become merely background noise. Our ancestors who paid attention to things that were out of place were more likely to survive and pass on this tendency to their offspring. Our ancestors who had more of a propensity to be content were less alert to threats and got eaten by the bear. "The brain is like Velcro for negative experiences and Teflon for positive ones—even though most of your experiences are probably neutral or positive" (Hanson, 2009, p.41). Our brains are designed to keep us alive, not happy.

Psychological studies have shown that people weigh negative information more heavily than positive information. The negativity bias can affect us so severely that it causes us to make blatantly irrational decisions. For instance, we avoid an option framed in terms of negative attributes, while we would gladly accept the same option when it is framed by its positive characteristics. Thus, people prefer flights that are on time eighty-eight percent of the time over flights that are late twelve percent of the time. In one study where researchers cooked ground beef for a taste test, participants who ate burgers that were described as "75% lean" rated them to be less greasy, leaner, and better in quality and taste than people who'd eaten identical burgers that were "25% fat."

Negative news coverage captures our attention, so news cycles globally focus on negative stories. How often have you heard a news anchor say, "In cities across America today, nothing in particular happened for millions of people." The news is always about what is unusual, often in a negative way. One researcher assessed the global demand for negative information in news cycles across seventeen countries. She found that the average human is physiologically more activated by negative news stories than positive ones (Soroka, 2019).

I remember a fellow who was referred to me because of uncontrolled hypertension. Various medications tried by his family physician did not seem to work. She referred him to a psychiatrist who also tried various medications, but none seemed to work. The psychiatrist referred him to me. I tried different relaxation techniques and none seemed to work. I knew I was missing something. I asked him to describe his typical day. He was recently retired, but had no particular plan for spending his time. His wife was still working full time and was gone during the day. He mostly puttered around the house doing various tasks but turned on cable news to "have company." He was a pleasant fellow, even-tempered and friendly. When he mentioned the news, I said something about a current event at the time. This friendly fellow suddenly became agitated and red-faced angry about politicians this and that and this issue and that issue. At that moment, I thought I had determined the problem. I asked him what kind of music he liked. Then I asked if he was willing to conduct an experiment. Would he be willing to turn off the news for two weeks and instead listen to his favorite music during the day for "company?" He agreed. Two weeks later and from then onward, his hypertension was resolved. The moral of the story? Be careful what you feed yourself. Too much negativity can be toxic.

According to reporting by the *Washington Post* (Oremus et al., 2021), Facebook programmed the algorithm that decides what people see in their news feeds to use the reaction emoji as a signal to push more emotional and provocative content—including content likely to make them angry. Facebook's internal documents reveal that, beginning in 2017, their ranking algorithm treated emoji reactions as more valuable than "likes." Posts that prompted many reaction emojis, especially anger, kept users online consuming content, which was vital to Facebook's business. Each user's feed reflects their interests. For a subset of highly partisan users, Facebook's algorithm can turn their feeds into echo chambers of divisive content and news of varying reputability that supports their outlook. The next time you spend fifteen minutes dressing down a "troll" on Facebook, understand that a software algorithm predetermined your actions. *Think about that for a minute.*

One study investigated whether there was a causal connection between adult social media use and subsequent increases in depressive symptoms. In this survey, thousands of individuals with minimal depressive symptoms who reported use of Snapchat, Facebook, or TikTok were more likely to report increased depressive symptoms on a later survey. These results suggest that certain social media use preceded the development of depressive symptoms (Perlis et al., 2021).

There are several theories about why social media has this effect on some people. One theory is the distortion that is created by selective posting. Imagine you had a bad day at work and feel lonely. You open Facebook and see post after post of people smiling, hanging out with friends, sharing vacation pics, reporting on their kid's most recent achievement, and so on. You think, *Everyone has a great life, and my day sucked.* Then you see the post from your crazy uncle about the latest conspiracy or political outrage. Before you know it, you have spent half an hour (or more) consuming a very distorted reality. Another theory suggests that the gradual increase in social media consumption in cyberspace may diminish the time spent engaging in actual activities in real space.

Research has shown a correlation between excessive social media use and increased rates of depression and anxiety. Studies have found that the more time individuals spent on social media, the more likely they were to report symptoms of depression (Kross et al., 2013) and that individuals who frequently compared themselves to others on social media had higher levels of depression and anxiety (Feinstein et al., 2013 (Feinstein, 2013)).

One such study followed a group of young adults over three years and found that higher levels of social media use at the beginning predicted significant depression and anxiety symptoms at the end of the study (Twenge et al., 2018). Another study followed a group of adolescents over two years and found that higher levels of social media use at the beginning of the study predicted greater depression symptoms at the end of the study, after adjusting for baseline depression symptoms (Leventhal et al., 2020). These studies suggest that social media use can be prospectively linked to depression and anxiety.

The moral of the story? To avoid the negativity bias, be careful of your consumption of news and social media. Be alert to exposing yourself to things that cultivate a negativity bias.

### Availability Heuristic

Amos Tversky and Daniel Kahneman's work (Tversky & Kahneman, 1973) helped generate insights about the *availability heuristic*. They described the availability heuristic as "whenever one estimates frequency or probability by the ease with which instances or associations could be brought to mind." In simpler terms, one guesses the likelihood that things happen by using easily recalled memories as a reference. We believe things that come to mind more easily to be far more common and accurate reflections of the real world.

Things like news reports can affect your estimate of how often things happen. If there are lots of news reports about terrorist attacks, we think about them often. They are usually horrible and dramatic, making them more easily recalled. This leads us to overestimate how often these events happen. You have more of a chance of being hit by lightning than directly experiencing a terrorist event, but the availability heuristic makes this seem not so. This cognitive bias can affect situations where we must thoughtfully evaluate risk, by leading us to over-estimate risk. This in turn causes us to act in a way that is not wise.

### Formulation Effects

Subtle aspects of how problems are posed, questions are phrased, and responses are elicited can substantially impact people's judgments (Fischhoff, 1980). For example, an action increasing one's chance of death from 1 in 10,000 to 1.3 in 10,000 is considered much riskier if the action were described as producing a thirty percent increase in annual mortality risk.

Another example is a study in which subjects were presented with detailed descriptions of two imaginary therapies for lung cancer. Subjects were given information regarding the effectiveness of the therapies in terms of either probability of surviving or dying (e.g., a sixty eight percent chance of surviving vs. a thirty two percent chance of dying). When a therapy was presented with the likelihood of dying, preferences dropped significantly over an identical therapy described in terms of probability of survival. The problem's presentation led to different preferences, even though the outcomes and probabilities were the same. The study found this effect to hold for both lay people and physicians (McNeil, 1982).

### Fundamental Attribution Error

Psychologist Lee Ross first proposed this cognitive bias in the early 1970s. People are constantly forming judgments about why other people behave the way they do. These judgments are called *attributions*. There are several ways these judgments can be biased. The fundamental attribution error refers to a biased tendency to attribute other people's behaviors to their inherent personalities or dispositions, rather than to situational factors. For example, if a coworker is often late for meetings, we might attribute the quality of being disorganized or irresponsible to them. We are less likely to attribute their tardiness to things like traffic during the commute or family or health issues. If a server is terse, we will think they have an unpleasant personality rather than consider that they might have a headache, or their boss just yelled at them, or their dog died this morning.

### Naïve Realism

This bias refers to our tendency to believe that we see the world objectively, without bias or influence from our perspective. If someone else thinks a different way, we view them as irrational, biased, or not well-informed. We expect others will come to the same conclusions so long as they are exposed to the same information and interpret it rationally. Recall the problem of perception explored in chapter 1. The fundamental problem with naïve realism is a somewhat self-centered arrogance. How I see it is how it is. It is more aligned with reality to be more humble concerning our perceptions. I recognize that I am a human being, flawed, and limited in my ability always to perceive things as they are. This is not the same as being perpetually filled with self-doubt, but a more realistic sense of knowing one's limitations. It is understanding that things aren't always as they appear.

### Discordant Knowing

A severe form of cognitive bias is *discordant knowing*. Discordant knowing is when someone is convinced they know something to be so because they *feel* it is. With discordant knowing, I *know* something is true. It does not matter what evidence there is to the contrary. It does not matter what experts say. I know it, and that is all that matters. This is a more extreme form of the cognitive distortion of emotional reasoning. In nine studies (N=3,277), Gollwitzer (2022) examined whether discordant knowing underlies fanaticism. Experimentally manipulating participants' views under this framework (e.g., "I am certain about X, but most other people think X is unknowable or wrong") heightened indicators of fanaticism, including aggression, determined ignorance, and wanting to join extreme groups in the service of these views.

More examples and explanations about cognitive biases and how they affect our decisions can be found in the book *Thinking, Fast and Slow* by Daniel Kahneman (2011). *The Drunkard's Walk* by Leonard Mlodinow (2009) explores how humans misjudge the effect that randomness has on our decision-makingarie. *Predictably Irrational* by Dan Ariely (2008) also explores how random and illogical thought processes influence our behavior. An excellent overview is found in the award-winning book *Thinking 101* by Yale professor Woo-kyoung Ahn (2022).

Understanding the various ways our perceptions can be distorted and biased is essential. If we don't do this, we risk being out of touch with things as they are and having these perceptions influence our feelings, actions, and how we conduct ourselves with others. As human beings, we are stuck with our perceptions. We are not fully capable of seeing things completely as they are. We are stuck in bodies that rely on our senses and minds to make sense of things. We only have access to a filtered version of reality. Since we live with this limitation in our day-to-day lives, it is good to have a humble view of our perceptions. *I am looking at things in a certain way, but I want to leave room for the possibility that I might be mistaken.*

## Reframing Thoughts vs. "Fighting" with Your Mind

When working with your thoughts, it is important not to set up a dynamic where you are "fighting" with your own thoughts. It is crucial to be a good observer of your thoughts. Notice what thoughts you are having. What put them in motion? Are the thoughts causing you to suffer from anxiety, depression, or anger? If I notice I am experiencing a thought that is not useful, a natural impulse is to try to "push the thought away." This is an interesting phrase. What does it mean to "push" a thought, and where exactly is "away?"

The more I "push" a thought away, the more the mind "pushes back." In a fight with your mind, your mind will usually be the victor. For this reason, it is better to *observe* rather than *fight*.

Take a few minutes to conduct a brief experiment. Close your eyes and take a breath or two. Imagine a pink elephant. Bring forth the image as clearly as you can. Now, imagine you have been told that thoughts about pink elephants are bad and it is vital that you push the thought away. Go ahead, push. What do you notice? Did the pink elephant vanish? No? Then try harder! What do you notice?

The more you fight to push away the pink elephant, the more it returns to front and center, even more energetically. The reason for this is that our minds are not wired for negation. As soon as I think, *I won't think about a pink elephant,* it's too late. I have already thought about it as an object I was not going to think about. This is a loop that I just get caught in over and over.

Now let's change the experiment. As before, bring forth the image of the pink elephant. This time, you will not fight with your mind. You observe that your mind is now thinking about a pink elephant. Rather than push the image away, gently hold on to it in your awareness. What do you notice? You probably notice that you can successfully hold onto the image for a moment or so, and then something happens. Your mind moves. The image of the pink elephant morphs, perhaps into a regular elephant, and then thoughts of a circus, elephants eating peanuts at the circus, and then peanut butter. Before you know it, you notice you are mulling over things you want to remember to get at the grocery store. When we gently observe, the mind naturally wants to move on to the next thing.

One more experiment modification. This time you again call forth the pink elephant. You remember those pink elephant thoughts are not useful. Instead of pushing the pink elephant away, you ask yourself what a useful thought is. For our experiment, you may decide that an image of a fluffy bunny is useful. Now focus your awareness on the bunny. You are not pushing the pink elephant away. You are merely directing your awareness toward the bunny. If your mind drifts, you may gently bring it back to the bunny if doing so is beneficial.

It is important when examining thoughts to be a good observer. Avoid judging your thoughts harshly. Harsh judgments are just more thoughts. When anchored in observer mode, I can be more thoughtful about my thoughts, the feelings they evoke, and whether it is wise to act on them. Sometimes simply observing is enough. Sometimes the work is to reframe the thought, but this is not the same as fighting with my thoughts. A reframe is merely observing a thought that is not useful and replacing it with a more useful one that aligns with Right Understanding. This is like focusing on the bunny instead of the pink elephant.

## Abnormal Thoughts

We understand now that some thoughts can result from a mental illness, an abnormality in the brain that disrupts psychological factors. We have a mind, but our mind lives in a brain. Sometimes the brain suffers from damage or disease, which affects how the mind functions.

An example of this is obsessive-compulsive disorder (OCD). One characteristic of OCD is experiencing unwanted thoughts (obsessions) that create anxiety and lead to overwhelming urges to engage in irrational actions (compulsions) to ease the anxiety. The obsessions and compulsive rituals reinforce each other to the point that the person uses a considerable amount of mental energy in managing them. The obsessive thoughts are experienced as not wanted and not part of the self. The technical term is *ego-dystonic*. The person suffering from OCD agrees the thoughts are irrational, but they are nonetheless overpowering.

There are several ways that this disorder can manifest. One common presentation is contamination fears. Here, the person might have an intrusive, unwanted thought that, after touching a public doorknob, they contracted a cancer virus. The individual knows there is no such thing as a cancer virus on doorknobs but cannot get this thought out of their head no matter how hard they try. They feel compelled to wash their hands in a compulsive ritual, sometimes repeatedly, to ease the anxiety associated with the irrational, obsessive thought. Other common presentations are checking OCD, counting OCD, need for symmetry, and fear of losing control.

What all these different forms of OCD have in common is an irrational unwanted thought that is experienced as ego-dystonic and a compulsive ritual in response to that thought. OCD is currently best understood as a mental illness related to abnormal functioning in the brain. It is not so much a psychological problem of the mind, but rather a brain disorder that affects psychological functioning.

What is one to do if one's brain is affecting psychological well-being? How can the Eightfold Path or CBT techniques work if the fundamental problem is brain functioning? We have a mind, but it exists in a brain. What are we supposed to do if our brain is not functioning correctly? These are excellent questions. It turns out that the influence can go both directions. My brain can affect how I function or feel psychologically. However, my mind and actions can affect my brain and how my brain functions.

The CBT treatment for OCD involves a cognitive reframing of the experience and exposure and response prevention (ERP). ERP involves exposure to the cue associated with the obsessive thought ("exposure"), and then letting the anxiety be fully experienced without trying to mitigate the anxiety through the compulsive ritual ("response prevention"). For example, with the contamination OCD example, the individual would purposely touch public doorknobs but resist the urge to wash their hands afterward. They would repeat this until the anxiety dissipated in the presence of the cue.

Research has shown that ERP treatment for OCD can be effective to reduce symptoms and lead to changes in brain activity (Bhagwagar, 2020; Chau, 2017). Several studies have found mindfulness practices and meditation to also be a very effective intervention for OCD (Wahl, 2013; Hertenstein, 2012; Hanstede 2008; see also chapter 10). Even though OCD has well-documented abnormal brain functioning, it nonetheless responds favorably to CBT techniques.

Some studies have suggested that mindfulness-based practices may benefit individuals with schizophrenia by helping to reduce symptoms such as psychosis, anxiety, and depression. One such study found that an eight-week mindfulness-based intervention (MBI) significantly reduced symptoms of psychosis, anxiety, and depression and improved the overall quality of life in individuals with schizophrenia. The study also found at a six-month follow-up that the effects of the MBI were sustained (Fjorback et al., 2011).

The point of discussing these mental health disorders is to understand that we all have a mind, but our mind lives in a brain. Some people have brain-based mental health disorders that can affect their thoughts. It is important to understand this and to realize that medication is sometimes needed to address the brain abnormality and create homeostasis. It is also important to know that the influences can go in both directions. My brain can affect my mind, but my mind can also affect my brain in desirable ways. This is well-documented by the influence of CBT and mindfulness-based practices on brain functioning.

## The Path Forward . . .

In this chapter, we explored the relationship between thoughts and suffering. As long as our thoughts reflect our seeing things as they are, our suffering will be reduced. We explored that within both the Buddhist and CBT frameworks, cultivating useful thoughts is essential for cultivating well-being within ourselves and others. We explored many examples of ways our thoughts can be distorted and out of alignment with how things are, based on learning and, to some extent, "hardwiring." These examples remind us to take a humble perspective about our perceptions. We can practice cultivating Right Thought by practicing compassionate thoughts of loving-kindness toward others and using various methods to actively correct distorted thinking.

Take some time to consider something that is currently causing some stress in your life. Is there anything that you notice about your thoughts related to this stress? Did you explore the event using the 3-column technique? If so, what did you notice.

Right Understanding and Right Thinking are the Buddhist foundations of wisdom. If we start with a foundation of wisdom, we will conduct ourselves ethically, which promotes harmony in our relationships with others and within ourselves. In the next chapter, we will explore how the wisdom of Right Understanding and Right Thinking is reflected in Right Speech toward others. And we will explore ways of improving our practice in this area.

# Part III

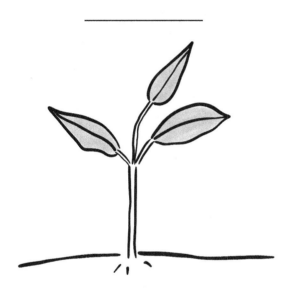

# Cultivating
an Ethical Path

# 5

# RIGHT
# SPEECH

*"Always speak the truth. Just don't always be speaking it."*
*– Grandma Jones*

# Buddhism and Right Speech

Right Speech refers to speaking in a way that is beneficial, truthful, and non-harmful to oneself and others. This includes refraining from lying, gossiping, harsh language, and divisive speech. Instead, the practice fosters open, honest communication that promotes understanding and compassion. It also encourages one to be mindful of the impact of one's words on others and to communicate with the intention of bringing about peace and harmony.

When I was younger, I remember conversing with my parents about their experiences in life. I asked what they thought the "secret" of a good marriage was. They had been happily married for over fifty-five years. My mother paused thoughtfully and replied, "I think talking is important. Some people don't talk when they should." After another pause she continued, "I think it is also important to know when not to talk. Some people talk when maybe they shouldn't." I'll leave that there for a moment—old-school wisdom.

Even though something might be true, said kindly, and thought to be helpful, it might not be the right time to speak. Knowing when and when not to speak is the secret to a happy marriage (and a good life). One of my mother's favorite sayings was "Always speak the truth. Just don't always be speaking it." This insight about being mindful of one's speech has always stayed with me. Not everything that is true needs to be spoken. The Buddha also talked about the importance of the timing of speech.

The great Sufi poet Rumi described this in a useful way: "Before you speak, let your words pass through three gates. When you arrive at the first gate, ask yourself, 'Is it true?' At the second gate, ask, 'Is it kind?' At the third gate, ask, 'Is it necessary or useful?'"

Rumi and Grandma Jones were saying similar things. Be thoughtful about your speech. Words are powerful and can impact others in the same way as our actions. So, before we speak, we can ask ourselves some reflective questions. *Am I saying something true? If it is not true, why am I thinking about saying it? Is my ego operating, am I defensive, or am I trying to manipulate in a way that affects the other party negatively?*

Next, why would I say something unkindly? I can share something brutally honest but say it in a way that strives to be kind. Is it kind to be "brutally" honest? What is the point of being "brutal?" Again, is my ego driving my actions?

At the last gate I must ask myself, *Do circumstances insist that saying this is necessary? Will the other party find what I have to say helpful?* If the answer is no, then I may want to resist speaking. Not everything that is true needs to be spoken aloud. Often the truth speaks for itself without any help from me. I might have something to say that is true, yet realize the other person would not benefit from my saying it.

Like the other practices of the Eightfold Path, Right Speech is not a stand-alone practice. We can see how Right Understanding leads to Right Thought, which leads to Right Speech. If we look at things incorrectly, engage in distorted thoughts as a result, and put those distorted thoughts into speech, we may say and do things that are hurtful, hateful, or cause division and suffering.

Alternatively, if we look at things clearly and in a way that reflects wise understanding, we will have clear thoughts and wise speech. Right Speech is, again, "right" in the sense of having the "right" key for a lock. What is effective and skillful? It isn't just about acting in a way that makes you a "good" person. It's about the most effective, compassionate, and genuine way to communicate and interact with other people.

Engaging in "wrong" speech creates problems that are not congruent with the Buddhist path. When receiving "wrong" speech, people get upset with you or don't believe you any longer because you've been less than truthful, or your idle talk causes ill will among others. The agitation that wrong speech elicits interferes with the practice of calming our minds. Wrong speech is often motivated by selfishness. Our preoccupation with our ego leads to a self-centered mindset that can cause our speech to be dishonest, inconsiderate, judgmental, or harsh. Practicing Right Speech requires us to let go of our ego and its preoccupations.

The Buddha taught that paying attention to how you express yourself verbally is essential to the practice. Our speech influences other people, and we care about that unless we are ignorantly bound to our own ego. On the positive side, our speech can convey love and support for others on their journey. Alternatively, on the negative side, our speech may trigger defensiveness or anger in others, or demoralize or confuse them. What we say to others has a powerful influence on our thinking and can reinforce positive or negative patterns of behavior.

Thich Nhat Hanh (1998) said, "Deep listening is the foundation of Right Speech. If we cannot listen mindfully, we cannot practice Right Speech. No matter what we say, it will not be mindful because we'll be speaking only our own ideas and not in response to the other person."

Right Speech refers to speaking in truthful, kind, and compassionate ways and avoiding speech that is harmful or hurtful to oneself or others. You might apply Right Speech in several ways in the context of mental health issues. For example, by being honest about your emotions and experiences and avoiding deception that can erode trust in relationships and harm your well-being. Gossip, criticism, and other forms of harmful or hurtful communication can also damage relationships. Damaged relationships can exacerbate mental health issues. It is important for mental health to speak kindly and compassionately, using gentle, supportive, and encouraging words while avoiding harsh or critical language. Right Speech can facilitate mental health by giving full attention to others when speaking without judgment or distraction. Active listening can help you build trust and connection in relationships and a sense of mutual understanding. It is also important to talk to yourself in kind, supportive, and encouraging ways and to avoid negative self-talk that can worsen mental health issues.

By applying Right Speech, you can develop greater self-awareness and cultivate positive relationships, which can help you reduce stress, anxiety, and other mental health symptoms. You can build trust, foster deeper connections, and promote emotional well-being by speaking truthfully, kindly, and compassionately.

## CBT and Right Speech

From a CBT perspective, Right Speech (speech that is truthful, kind, and helpful) can be seen as the importance of developing healthy communication skills. In this perspective, Right Speech can be cultivated by learning to recognize and challenge communication habits that contribute to emotional distress and psychological problems.

In a CBT framework, we learn to use assertive communication techniques, such as expressing needs and boundaries clearly and directly while also being respectful of others. By learning to communicate more effectively, we develop healthier relationships and reduce interpersonal conflicts, thus improving mental health and well-being.

## Active Listening vs. Passive Listening

Not all listening is the same. Often when listening to someone else speak, we *listen passively*. We may hear their words, but we are not listening mindfully. We may only listen for the pause in their speech to say the words we were listening to in our minds. This happens often in heated conversations. The other problem with passive listening is that while we might be listening and can even repeat what the other person just said, they may not *feel listened to.*

If you find the other party often repeats themselves, making the same point in slightly different ways, they might feel you are not listening because you are not giving any clues that you understand what they are saying.

*Active listening* is when we are very mindful while the other person is speaking. We pay attention to the meaning of what they are saying and attend to nuance. We avoid interrupting. We ask on-point questions to understand better. We avoid questions that are argumentative and only make a point instead of developing understanding. We occasionally paraphrase what we hear to check if our understanding is correct. For example: "What I hear you say is . . . Is that the main point?" When people engage in active listening, each party is more likely to feel understood, and feeling understood is the basis of intimacy and harmonious relationships.

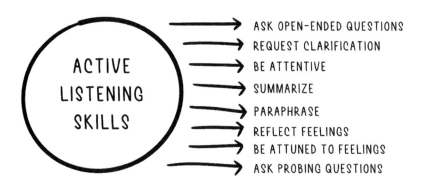

*Figure 9: Active Listening Skills*

## The Four Horsemen

John Gottman is a psychologist who conducted several studies examining the differences between distressed and satisfied couples (Gottman J., 2000; Gottman & Gottman, 2008). He found that four specific behaviors captured much of the difference between satisfied and distressed couples. Gottman called them the "Four Horsemen" (after the Four Horsemen of the Apocalypse in the Bible), because if they are not corrected, they predict "endings." These four behaviors are criticism, defensiveness, contempt, and stonewalling. Fortunately, each of the Four Horsemen has a corresponding "antidote," or the thing to do instead of the horseman behavior. The antidotes are correlated with increased relationship satisfaction.

I have found the Four Horsemen framework to be very useful in my work with couples, and over time discovered that is also very helpful for almost any pairing of people, such as parents-children, employee-supervisor, supervisor-subordinate, or friend-friend.

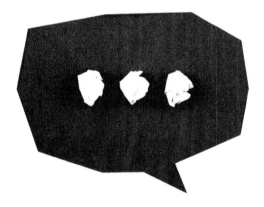

### *#1 Criticism*

The first horseman is CRITICISM. Criticism is when you explain to the other person how they need to improve as a human being, what is wrong with them, what they did not do right, and so on. It usually takes the form of a "you-statement." A you-statement usually begins with the word "you," followed by the critique. For example, "You know what your problem is? You always this, you never that . . ." Usually, the criticizer feels very justified and self-righteous in their criticism. After all, they are trying to help the other party to be a better human being.

Criticisms often have difficulty passing through Rumi's "three gates." While there might be some truth to the complaint, criticisms usually omit or distort certain things. Criticisms often are voiced unkindly and in a way that is unnecessary or not useful to the person receiving them.

Sometimes people don't realize they are being critical. They might claim, "I'm just saying how I feel," as if that makes everything okay. A common mistake is to convince myself I am using an "I-statement," but when I say, "I feel you always this or you never that," the sentence starts with the word I, but the communication itself is critical.

Even if I use a kind and measured tone of voice, but the heart of what I am saying is critical, I will probably experience a negative reaction from the other party.

### Instead of Criticism—Express a Need

We must first understand that criticism is a poorly expressed need. The other party usually responds to the criticism instead of the under-lying need. It's like putting a present inside a prickly box. The reaction is to the box, not the contents. I may be hurt or disappointed that my gift was rejected when the other person is rejecting the packaging. This is how criticisms often lead to my needs getting lost in the exchange.

Expressing a need is usually more fruitful than expressing a feeling. All someone can do with a feeling is try to empathize. There is nothing wrong with empathy, but it is limited. Expressing a need connects us to the outside world and provides something that the other person can perhaps relate to.

I am not self-contained. I am interdependent with the world outside of me, and to be happy and well I need things from that world. When you feel a negative emotion, the homeostasis of your well-being is disturbed. For example, you don't feel content because you are thirsty. You believe a drink of water will restore you to contentment. This basic idea is true for other emotional needs. If you can define what would restore you to a content state in terms that are doable and observable, you will make a good expression of need. It is helpful to practice translating feelings into needs

People often voice their needs in overly abstract terms, such as "respect me more," "I need more love and affection," or "I need more help." These types of abstract phrases might generate a picture in the other person's mind that differs from the one in your mind. Ask yourself, "If the other person were to meet this need, what that would look like?" Then express your need in doable and observable terms. You can ask the same question if someone expresses a need to you in abstract terms, to encourage them to be more specific.

Remember that in the Buddhist framework, it is essential to be careful about the connection between desire and suffering. *Is my need doable and observable? Is it considered with loving-kindness toward the other party? Is the need arising from some preoccupation of my ego?* It is good to express healthy needs in a loving way. It is also good to check whether your need reflects a wholesome desire.

## #2 Defensiveness

Usually, when people receive criticism, they respond by becoming defensive or arguing the merits of the criticism. While the criticism might be technically true, the other party will assert that they had righteous motives, or that the complaint is exaggerated or leaves out something important. Defensiveness communicates to the other party: "What you just said has no merit."

Now if we go back to the criticizer's point of view, they are thinking: *Wait a minute. I don't say things that have no merit. It's probably because you don't understand. Let me repeat myself, give you more examples of your shortcomings, or say it louder* (we all know things are truer if said louder).

The person on defense may then attack with criticism of their own, eliciting defensiveness in their conversational partner. This back and forth can continue until emotions get stronger. This escalation then leads to the third horseman.

### Instead of Defensiveness—Find the Merit, Then Find the Need

The antidote to defensiveness has two parts. Both are important. If the other party is criticizing you, they are trying to express a need, but doing it poorly. The object is to find the need. To get there, we first need to find the merit in the criticism.

Finding the merit in the criticism does not mean you agree with the criticizer entirely and wholeheartedly. It comes from understanding that complaints are often exaggerated, leave out important aspects of the problem, and are sometimes self-serving or unfair. However, there is usually a kernel of truth. By merely acknowledging the truth of that kernel, you open the door to finding the need. Don't get side-tracked and debate the merits of the criticism—that merely gives the horseman energy. If there is truth in the criticism, it is wise to accept it and adjust your actions. If the criticism has no truth, then there is no reason to become defensive.

When considering the merits of the criticism, remember this important question: "Do you want to be right or happy?" If you want to be right, by all means, argue the merits until you win. Just be advised that this will probably be at the expense of your happiness and the other party's happiness.

After you acknowledge the merit of the criticism, ask the other party what they need. What would help them be happy and well? What do they need in the present moment? If you were to meet this need, what would that look like?

### #3 Contempt

Contempt is a feeling of general hostility or disgust toward the other party. We see them in globally negative terms. Sometimes we can disagree with someone and still feel love or affection toward them. With contempt, there is a loss of perspective, and of love. One forgets the good qualities of the other party and the good motives they have most of the time. Contempt can be expressed subtly, such as rolling your eyes or communicating disrespect, or more directly, such as shouting or name-calling. In the Buddhist framework, when I feel contempt, I am caught in the poison of hatred. It is hard to communicate effectively when under the influence of this poison, because I come from a place of ego rather than loving-kindness.

When all the horsemen are galloping around, it often leads to elevated emotional arousal. When this arousal becomes high enough, it causes *flooding*. Flooding is when one experiences a deluge of stress chemicals along with the accompanying negative emotions of either anxiety or anger. This flooding then leads to the fourth horseman.

### Instead of Contempt—Keep Perspective

The hostility and disgust of the third horseman, contempt, often derive from a loss of perspective. When we think of the other party in globally negative terms, we lose sight of important things. What do I love and respect about them when I am not upset or angry? Can I call those aspects forward now? Why was this person at one time my friend? Am I personalizing this exchange and ignoring other factors influencing the other party? Keeping perspective requires us to practice mindfulness and see our reactions in context.

Another way to keep perspective is to assume neutral motives for the other party. We often get drawn into contempt when we attribute hostile intentions to others. For example, they forgot to pick up the item we asked them to, and we believe they did it intentionally. We make mistakes. We forget things. However, we usually have neutral motives. Try to keep that as your assumption when interacting with others.

It is hard to think of positive things when we are angry, anxious, or upset. So, prepare in advance. When you are calm, create a shortlist of what you love and respect about the other person. Then mentally rehearse this list until you can bring those aspects instantly to mind if suddenly put on the spot. This will help you to keep these things in mind under the stress of a disagreement.

## #4 Stonewalling

Stonewalling is when one party shuts down and withdraws from the conversation. They might physically withdraw by leaving the room or mentally withdraw by no longer taking part in the conversation. The "silent treatment" is a good example of stonewalling. About eighty percent of the time, it is men who stonewall. Men tend to experience conflict as more unpleasant in a visceral sense. Usually, things will be "chilly" for a few hours or sometimes days, then one party or the other will do something to break the ice. They then return to interacting normally. However, because what was being discussed was not resolved, it lies dormant as an open item likely to be drawn into the next disagreement. This can become a vicious cycle, where a conversation about anything quickly escalates into a conversation about all unresolved open items.

### Instead of Stonewalling—Pause, Repair, and Restart

Remember that stonewalling results from being flooded with negative emotions. Nobody does anything well when flooded. The first thing to do is to calm down a few notches. This might take a few seconds, hours, or a good night's sleep. It should not take longer than twenty-four hours. If it does, you might have another problem that must be addressed. Once you are calmer, then make repair.

Repair differs from saying you're sorry. Saying you're sorry often addresses the *content* of the disagreement. Repair addresses *how* we had the conversation. Repair might sound like this:

"You know that conversation we had this morning? I didn't like the way that went. I think my part in it was that I got pretty defensive when you were bringing up the issue. I also raised my voice, which probably wasn't helpful."

That's it. Just consider two or three ways in which you may have contributed to the conversation being a lousy one, and then own them. It's that simple. It's also powerful. Repair keeps a lousy conversation from contaminating the following conversation(s).

After making repair, you can attempt to restart the conversation without restarting the argument. If we take a break, calm down, and then try to restart the conversation without first making repair, there is a good chance we will again fall into an argument. Exchanges that end in stonewalling remain like dry kindling waiting to be reignited.

### The Four Horsemen and Their Antidotes

| THE HORSEMEN | THE ANTIDOTES |
|---|---|
| CRITICISM | EXPRESS A NEED |
| DEFENSIVENESS | FIND THE MERIT, THEN FIND THE NEED |
| CONTEMPT | KEEP PERSPECTIVE |
| FLOODING | PAUSE, REPAIR, RESTART |

## Toxic Phrases to Avoid

Toxic things are harmful, dangerous, or poisonous. They can injure or kill. Toxic phrases reflect "wrong" speech that is harmful to our relationships with others. Here are some examples of toxic phrases to practice avoiding:

*"I told you so."*

When we go through something difficult, we feel bad. If your partner is going through something difficult, why make them feel worse by reminding them that you told them this would happen? Better to use the opportunity to be supportive. Sometimes it is best to let reality speak for itself.

*"You need to . . ."*

It is arrogant and presumptuous to think we know what somebody else needs without them telling us. If you want to know what *I* need, ask me. Otherwise, you might be referring to what *you* need. Sometimes this phrase also implies there is a simple solution that the person is not seeing. Often, we struggle because many factors are pressing on us, and the situation in our mind does not seem amenable to a simple solution.

*"I know how you feel."*

It is common to use this phrase in casual conversation. We usually mean, "I know how I felt in a similar situation" or "I know how I imagine I would feel if I were in that situation." We never know how someone feels. We can only do our best to understand how they must feel. No two situations are identical, and no two people are identical in how they react to situations. Never presume you *know* how the other person feels. Sometimes it is better to simply ask: "How do you feel about that?"

*"It's not a big deal."*

This statement reflects the earlier discussion on understanding objective topics versus subjective ones. This statement takes something subjective and turns it into a blanket statement of fact. It may not be a big deal to you, but it is to me. The statement may be a well-intentioned effort to help the other person keep perspective. The problem is that it invalidates the person going through an emotionally charged situation. Better to validate how the person feels and explore ways to help them overcome the powerful emotions they are dealing with.

*"You're just like your father (or your mother, sister . . .)."*

Even if the other person behaved like that person for a moment, you would reduce them to a persistent negative trait. It is also a classic criticism (as are most phrases that start with "you"), so it is likely to evoke a defensive response. Rather than discussing the issues in terms of static traits, try to address the specific behavior and express whatever need you might have.

*"You always . . ." or "You never . . ."*

It is rarely the case that someone always does something or never does something. When frustrated, we exaggerate and unintentionally elicit a defensive response because of our all-or-nothing frame. "I don't always do that. Last Wednesday, I didn't." We likely mean to say that this behavior happens more than we would prefer, or that it would please us to see this behavior happen more often.

*"You're too sensitive." "You're overreacting."*
When someone is upset, and you blow them off by insisting they're "too sensitive" or "too emotional," you act as if you are the final judge of their feelings. Whenever we use the modifier "too," there is an implied anchor point or cut-off. This statement reflects a subjective viewpoint presented as fact.

*"Sorry."*
Don't say you're sorry. Say, "I apologize." Making an apology means taking action. It's more active and powerful. Plus, in common usage, we're skeptical of "sorry." Too many people use "sorry" as a weasel word to shut down the conflict and get out of genuinely apologizing.

*"Can't you just . . . ?"*
This phrase suggests that there's a simple solution to the problem and implies that the other person is deficient in not seeing it. It is a way of dismissing the other person's concerns or perspective. Often this toxic phrase will elicit a sarcastic thought like, *Wow, I wish I had thought of that.*

*"I'm just being honest."*
First, it is problematic to assert this. Why would you be anything other than honest? We sometimes use "honesty" as a shield to excuse being unkind or unhelpful. Ask yourself if the person is really going to benefit from your "honesty," or whether you are serving a need within yourself. Sometimes we are just trying to elevate ourselves. Remember Grandma Jones' suggestion: Always speak the truth. Just don't always be speaking it.

## Mission vs. Position

Sometimes, when speaking with someone, our challenge is finding a way to blend our needs. All too often, we approach these kinds of conversations as a contest. Any contest has a winner and a loser. "My needs versus your needs" creates conflict.

In the book *Getting to Yes*, the authors present an idea called "Mission vs. Position" (Fisher & Ury, 2006). The mission is *what* we want to accomplish. The position is my idea about *how* we should accomplish it. For example, we might have a shared mission that tonight we should have a pleasant evening together. My partner might adopt the position that we should do dinner and a movie to accomplish the mission. I might adopt the position that we go to the park and feed the ducks. Often conflict can arise because we get emotionally invested in our respective *positions* and need to remember the shared *mission.*

If I adopt a position about how things should be, and the other party assumes a contrary position, the more our egos get attached to our respective positions, the more the conflict escalates. We take the differences personally, causing our minds to close to alternatives. If we instead blend our needs, we will probably be able to discern creative solutions that address our concerns and keep our minds focused on the mission.

There is a Japanese martial art called aikido. In Japanese, *ai* means "harmony or love." *Ki* means "spirit, mind, or energy." *Do* means "path, journey, teaching, way." So, Ai-ki-do is the path of harmonizing energy. When an aikido practitioner meets an attack, the idea is not to meet force with force in a collision. The practice is to blend with the attack and dissipate the aggression harmlessly in a throw or pin. This idea of blending is a useful physical metaphor for dealing with interpersonal and verbal conflict. Am I arguing my point in trying to "win" the contest? Or am I doing my best to harmonize or blend my position with the other party's position?

Usually, our speech will be divisive and will generate ill will when we try to assert our needs at the expense of the other party's needs. Rarely are the needs truly mutually exclusive. When it seems they are, it is often the result of how we have framed the needs.

Try saying, "What do you need in this situation to be happy and well? If I met that need, what would that look like?" Paraphrase the other person's response to ensure you are actively listing and understanding correctly. Then express your perspective: "Okay, this is what I need to be happy and well. What are your ideas about how we might blend our needs?" The purpose of this structure is to maximize happiness for both parties. It will also reveal if the other person has no interest in your needs and is only interested in their own.

## Explaining "It"

Another form of speech to avoid is what I like to call explaining "It." This relates to the third gate in Rumi's framework: *Is what I am about to say necessary or thought to be helpful to the other party?* "It" refers to things that you usually don't have to explain to an average adult. For example, "When you call me vulgar names, it hurts my feelings," "When you mock me when I am telling you my needs, I feel bad," "You promised to do one thing and instead did another, and that damages my trust in you," and "Please don't deny things I saw with my own eyes."

"It" can refer to something I have already said twenty-five times before. When I often must repeat myself, the other person likely heard the message but disregarded it. Why will they finally get "It" on the twenty-sixth explanation? There's no point in trying to tell them yet again. Sometimes people who profoundly lack empathy or often reveal an absence of conscience simply don't understand.

## The Path Forward . . .

Our journey so far has explored the importance of seeing things as they are and having thoughts aligned with reality. If our understanding and thoughts reflect wisdom, then our speech will reflect that wisdom. It will be truthful and promote harmony. It will not be divisive and create ill-will. Our mission with Right Speech is to try to understand the other from a place of loving-kindness, to express our needs clearly, and to seek harmony.

Consider what part of your speech could you improve. What "gate" do I often disregard? Does my speech come from a place of Right Understanding and Right Thought? Do the "Horsemen" sometimes get away from me?

In the next chapter, we will explore how the wisdom of Right Understanding and Right Thought are reflected in our actions. We will examine how our actions can reduce suffering in ourselves and others, and how sometimes the right thing to do is counterintuitive.

# 6

# RIGHT ACTION

*"Right action is the art of moving through life with mindful steps, where every gesture becomes a brushstroke of compassion and wisdom."*
*- Thich Nhat Hanh*

# Buddhism and Right Action

Right Action refers to ethical conduct and behavior that aligns with Buddhism's principles, such as avoiding causing harm to others and living non-violence. This includes refraining from stealing, lying, and engaging in unhealthy relationships or actions. Right Action is an essential aspect of Buddhism, as it helps to cultivate inner peace and harmony with the world around us. It is also seen as a way to purify the mind and reduce negative karma.

When we discussed Right Speech, we noted how speech is powerful and can cause goodwill or harm. In this sense, knowing when not to speak and when to speak is essential. The same holds for Right Action. Sometimes Right Action involves restraint or simply not acting. Sometimes the right action is to do nothing. Sometimes it is acting with focused intention.

In Buddhism, karma refers to the law of cause and effect. Karma is where actions (good or bad) have consequences that can affect a person's current and future situation. Negative karma refers to harmful or unethical actions that can lead to adverse effects in the future. These actions can include causing harm to others, engaging in dishonest behavior, or living a life of selfishness and greed. Negative karma can manifest in suffering, difficulty, or problems in one's life. Actions that benefit oneself and others generate positive karma and can lead to good consequences in the future.

Right Action involves avoiding causing harm to others, whether physically, verbally, or mentally. This includes refraining from killing, stealing, or engaging in deceitful or harmful behavior, honoring one's promises and commitments, and being truthful in one's words and actions. It also includes not engaging in sexual misconduct, such as infidelity or exploitation, and refraining from using drugs or alcohol in a way that clouds the mind or leads to negative behavior. Right Action entails living a simple and modest lifestyle, avoiding greed and excessive consumption, working to promote peace and harmony in one's community, alleviating suffering and injustice, practicing generosity and compassion, and helping others in need.

It's important to note that Right Action is closely related to the other paths of Buddhism, and the actions considered "right" may vary depending on the individual and the context.

Knowing which actions will produce greater happiness, wisdom, and well-being and relieve suffering requires discernment that is dependent upon Right Understanding. Without understanding how things are, we can easily act in a way that we think will be productive, only to find it destructive. If we have Right Thought, we will tend to take Right Action. As mentioned before, "right" here refers to the sense of being the "right key for a lock" rather than a set of ethical rules.

Sometimes our actions are motivated by wrong intentions of desire, ill-will, and causing harm. Right Action involves letting go of longing, practicing goodwill, and holding an attitude of harmlessness.

The monk Ledi noted that someone might claim to be a Buddhist and even have Right Understanding, but that does not necessarily mean they will put it into practice. "To know the good does not mean one will do it. All of one's book learning will not change harmfulness into loving-kindness. Only actual application and practice will result in Right Action" (Ledi, 1977).

The Buddha spoke of Right Action in three categories: 1. abstaining from killing, 2. abstaining from taking what is not given freely, and 3. abstaining from sexual misconduct.

Killing by accident is not accompanied by any degree of negative karma, as there was no intent to kill or harm. The motive for killing carries grave weight, and killing from a motive of greed, hatred, or ignorance is the worst kind. There is a karmic difference between stepping on a bug and enjoying stepping on a bug.

The antidote for abstaining from taking life is loving-kindness and compassion for all sentient beings—identifying with all beings with heartfelt sympathy and wishing for their welfare. Right Thought means goodwill, harmlessness, and concern for others. When we feel respect and loving-kindness for others, we cannot harm others (Holmes, 2017).

The second aspect of Right Action concerns abstaining from taking what is not given—in other words, not stealing. On this point, the Buddha's message is clear. Refrain from removing or appropriating anything without the owner's consent, either by physical effort or by inciting another to do so. We should not take with bad intent any possession of another person. It is equally wrong to withhold from others what should be rightfully theirs.

Similarly, stealing, robbery, snatching, fraudulence, and deceit carry negative karmic weight and hinder spiritual development. The antidote is honesty, respecting the property and rights of others, being content with one's livelihood, showing generosity of heart, and not coveting the wealth and possessions of others (Holmes, 2017).

Abstaining from taking what someone does not give freely also applies to nonmaterial things. If we argue, insist, or manipulate to get our way at the expense of someone else's suffering, this is like stealing. We are taking something from the other person that was not given freely. Try to adopt an attitude of only accepting what is given freely.

The third aspect of Right Action is to abstain from sexual misconduct. The Buddha tells us to refrain from any conduct in sensual pleasures that will cause pain to others. We do not derive sexual misconduct from some moral prescription. As noted before, "right" is derived from its observed effect. Does it cause suffering in the other party? Does it cause suffering in others involved? Does it cause suffering that detracts from one's path? The opposite of desiring somebody as an object to fulfill sensual desires is to see that person as they are—a human being worthy of care, regard, and compassion—and to feel loving-kindness toward that person that transcends the limits of mere grasping and desire.

In a Buddhist framework, it is essential to monitor the effects derived from one's actions. The Buddha once taught a disciple about reflecting on actions and assessing whether they are skillful. He advised asking oneself *before* acting, whether that action would cause suffering in oneself, others, or both? If so, I should resist the action. If I determine the consequences will benefit me, others, or both, then I may proceed. He also advised repeating the questions *during* the action. Is what I am doing now causing suffering in myself or others? If so, then stop. If not, then proceed. Finally, *after* the action is complete, what impact do I observe on myself and others? If the action resulted in pleasant effects for myself and others, I should continue practicing that action. If not, I should avoid that action in the future.

When is the best time to assess whether an action is skillful? The answer is *before* the action, *during* the action, and *after* the action. Sometimes we get attached to original intentions and stay the course, ignoring direct experience that contradicts the wisdom of continuing the action. The idea is to be mindful and adjust based on experience. This is being skillful.

The ethical aspect of Right Action is to avoid doing things that create suffering. This applies to self and others. If I lie, cheat, steal, and behave unethically, I will cause suffering in others and myself. Right Action applies to any behavior that cultivates a feeling of well-being, loving-kindness, and peacefulness, while avoiding those that cause suffering.

# CBT and Right Action

In the previous chapters, we explored how CBT can help with Right Understanding by guiding us to understand the limits of our perception and not be deceived by concepts related to self. We also explored how CBT relates to identifying and correcting distorted thoughts and how we can use CBT concepts to interact more effectively with others via our speech.

CBT focuses on the connections between a person's thoughts, feelings, and behaviors. It can be related to the Buddhist concept of Right Action, as both focus on aligning thoughts and actions with ethical principles and behaviors that avoid causing suffering in ourselves or others.

A CBT framework encourages cultivating Right Action through mindful behavior. By becoming more aware of our actions and their impact on ourselves and others, we can recognize and challenge behaviors that contribute to emotional distress and psychological problems. Right Action might also include identifying goals that align with one's values and taking small steps toward those goals daily. One can develop a sense of purpose and direction by taking consistent action toward meaningful goals.

CBT is also about changing our behaviors to be more effective and skillful and to reduce stress or suffering. Often, behavior change can be counterintuitive. Our instinct might tell us to do one thing, but what is actually effective is another. People often intuitively gravitate toward two methods of coping with negative emotions:

1.  **Distraction.** The first method is finding something to focus on that distracts us from whatever troubles us. This method can work for what we might call everyday troubles. However, its limitation is that the thing I use to distract myself must have more engaging energy than the thing troubling me. If it doesn't, then the distraction method doesn't work as well.

2. **Waiting.** The second common method is to wait for the negative feeling to run out of energy. This, too, can work, eventually. However, eventually can be hours or days, or even longer.

In the Buddhist framework, we asked when is the best time to assess whether an action is skillful. The answer was *before* the action, *during* the action, and *after* the action. An extension of this idea is often used in a CBT approach. I like to call it paying attention to the "cusp." Part of mindfulness is noticing movements in our mind and the factors that might cause them. I may notice that I was in a positive mood yesterday, and today in the evening, I am depressed or anxious. Between yesterday and now, there was a shift from one state to another. If I reflect on exactly when I noticed the shift beginning, I am then in a good position to examine the situational or mental conditions that shifted along with the mood.

The common approach of CBT and the Eightfold Path is to actively examine the source of our suffering and then adjust to correct it. So far, we have discussed how suffering can come from not understanding things correctly. We reviewed how thoughts can be a source of negative emotions. We also have explored how our speech can create ill will with others and how to adjust our speech to avoid this problem. Let's now explore some common ways our actions may unintentionally make things worse in four significant areas: depression, anxiety, anger, and sleep. We will then explore actions that are more effective but sometimes counterintuitive.

## Depression

Clinical depression can affect people in a variety of ways. It is often marked by a persistent sad mood or diminished ability to respond to pleasurable events. Sleep, appetite, concentration, and energy levels can all feel "off." Also very common is a distinct lack of motivation to do things you might normally do. The thought of doing most anything is met with a sense of "meh."

A low mood will cause a decrease in activity level. This may start subtly, such as skipping exercise, declining an invitation to go out with friends, or not engaging in a hobby. Research has shown that this shrinking activity level will then cause a further worsening in mood. In general, the less active we are, the fewer opportunities there are to experience positive things that might push our mood in a positive direction.

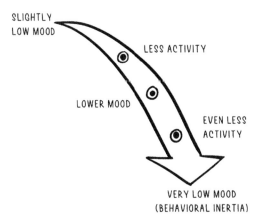

SLIGHTLY
LOW MOOD

LESS ACTIVITY

LOWER MOOD

EVEN LESS
ACTIVITY

VERY LOW MOOD
(BEHAVIORAL INERTIA)

*Figure 10: Activity Level and Mood*

Now, remember that a lowered mood causes a shrinking of activity level, which causes a further lowering of mood. This further reduced mood then causes a further shrinking of activity level. Variables that work this way bounce (Rethorst CD, 2009) off each other. They are both cause and effect. What then often evolves is a vicious spiral: low mood —> lowered activity level—> lower mood —> even lowered activity level —> even lower mood, and so on. People with depression may notice that the range of things they currently do compared to a few months before occupies a much smaller circle. This is described as becoming *mood dominant*, meaning that our mood dictates our decisions about what we want to do.

The bad news is that vicious spirals are, well, vicious. This activity-mood spiral can cause an oppressive feeling of inertia. The good news about vicious spirals is that they move in both directions. Therefore, if the activity level increases, the mood will increase, leading to still higher activity levels and a further rise in mood.

The difficulty is that with depression, when the spiral approaches the bottom, there is a great deal of behavioral inertia. At that point, a person with depression may not feel like doing anything, even taking a shower or getting out of bed.

The key here is the word "feel." We often consult our feelings when deciding what to do. We ask ourselves: *Hmm . . . I wonder if I feel like going to work out today?* If my feelings are functioning normally, this is a perfectly reasonable question to ask myself. Most days, I might feel like it, and occasionally I might not. The problem with depression is that it is a mood disorder. My mood is not operating normally. When

I am in a state that is mood dominant, anytime I ask my mood about doing something, the answer will always be no. I wait until the proper feeling is present, but it never seems to come.

## Override Low Inertia with Activity

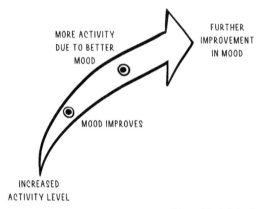

*Figure 11: Activity Level and Mood 2*

If we understand this process, we can use this understanding to do an intellectual override of the pattern. The principle to apply is "Do first. Let the feeling catch up." You let go of the expectation that the proper feeling or motivation must be present before you engage in an activity. You don't ask your mood, because it's not working properly. You do the activity first, *despite not feeling motivated.* You think, *Of course, I don't feel like it. I have depression. But I will do it anyway because I understand how the spiral works.* You cannot, through force of will, change your mood when suffering from depression, but you can initiate action, which then influences your mood in a positive direction. In this case, Right Action is counterintuitive.

There are many activities I might decide to do. One that allows you to see this dynamic is exercise. Exercise is very beneficial for depression. One meta-analysis found that exercise significantly lowered depression scores in participants, compared to those who didn't exercise (Rethorst et al., 2009).

Exercise does not have to be a six-mile run. It can be thirty minutes of simple walking. If I walk even though I don't feel like it, I will be more motivated to do other things afterward. Activities don't have to be a big deal or glamorous. Simple pleasures like a walk in nature, playing with a pet, or sitting in a park will do. Engaging in a hobby you have not done in a while is also good. Also beneficial are tasks that provide a sense of accomplishment, like making a meal, gardening, or finishing that small project you have been avoiding.

A tool that often helps with depression is activity scheduling. With this behavioral treatment for depression (Lewinsohn et al., 1969) instead of relying on fluctuations in mood to dictate what you do, schedule a variety of activities you might normally do at various times during the week. You might plan things like walking at a specific time each day, or practicing guitar, or watching a movie. You might schedule lunch with a friend you haven't seen in a while. Think about activities that were normal for you to do when you were not struggling with depression and put them on the schedule. Once you have your schedule, instead of asking whether you are in the mood (of course you're not; you have depression), you ask yourself, *What time is it?* and then do whatever is on the schedule—despite the mood of the moment. Give the appointment with yourself the same status you might give a doctor's appointment or business meeting. This is how we apply the "Do first. Let the feeling catch up" principle. When you get the hang of activity scheduling, you will be on your way to turning the spiral around and overcoming part of the inertia that keeps you trapped in depression.

## Anxiety and Avoidance

Fear is a natural response to physical threats. It has survival value. If a bear suddenly appears and wants to eat you, it is vital to mobilize the biological processes to fight the bear effectively or run away. This stress response is sometimes called the *fight-or-flight response*. It is a useful response, even in modern life, to *physical* threats.

However, anxiety is a *conditioned fear*. Our brains can make associations between things that are *actual* threats and things that are *related to* threats. In our bear example, let's imagine our first encounter with the bear is in a pretty meadow with flowers and butterflies. The bear comes after me, but I successfully run away though terrified of being nearly eaten by a bear. The next time I am out searching for food, I suddenly realize I am in the same meadow where I encountered the bear. Immediately I feel anxious. Not in response to the bear. It's not here now. I feel anxious in response to the meadow, flowers, and butterflies that I now associate with the bear. Flowers are not dangerous. But they now make me nervous because I associate them with the bear, which *is* dangerous. Our ancestors who could make these associations were more likely to survive. Those who did not tended to have further unpleasant encounters with bears.

So, anxiety has an evolutionary benefit that we should first honor as we try to understand our struggles with anxiety. At times the brain's tactic of making associations becomes maladaptive. If I have a panic attack in a grocery store, I will start associating the fear response with the grocery store, and I will then avoid that grocery store to manage the anxiety. Pretty soon, any grocery store will cue anxiety, so I avoid them. Then any store that is like a grocery store will have the same effect, and so on.

Evolution designed us to be hardwired to respond to anxiety by moving away from (escaping or avoiding) things that cue anxiety. This response can feel so strong that our survival seems to depend on moving away. We often feel the threat viscerally in our bodies as elevated arousal, preparing us for a physical threat. With generalized anxiety, the anxious response is to *psychological* rather than *physical* threats. Even though no physical threat is present, our brain responds as though it is.

This fight-or-flight reaction happens in the middle part of our brain, which operates more automatically. This part of the brain is simply reactive. It doesn't think things through. That is why it can be difficult to "reason" with anxiety. Our frontal lobe is the part of our brain that reasons things out. That is why we sometimes experience a duality. One part of my brain is saying a bear will eat me, while another part is aware there is no danger. This contradiction can make us feel a little crazy. It is real that the situation is benign. It is also real that I feel like a bear is going to eat me. Part of the reason people often deal with anxiety by avoidance is that it works really well. If something makes me anxious, I escape from the situation or avoid it altogether—*Whew! I feel much better!* My anxiety is almost immediately relieved. However, I am paying a penalty for that relief. Each time I escape or avoid, I strengthen the anxiety cue. My actions are making the problem worse.

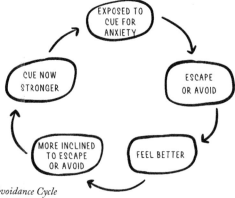

*Figure 12: Anxiety Avoidance Cycle*

## Exposing Our Worries

Most successful treatments for anxiety involve some form of exposure. Exposure involves systematically moving *toward* the situation or thing that is cueing anxiety. When you expose yourself to a conditioned fear, you will experience the level of fear corresponding to the cue's current strength. We have noted before that mother nature has hardwired us to have a default response be to escape or avoid. What happens if I override that default response and stay exposed to the cue?

If we maintain exposure, the fight-or-flight part of our brain will begin firing in concert with the sensory processing center that keeps track of our location (e.g., I am in an elevator, I am near a snake, I am in the grocery store). The anxiety signal tells us: "Get out! Danger!" If our actions instead say, "Nah, I'm good. I will stay here because I learned all about this in therapy," the fight-or-flight part of the brain will then increase the anxiety level, telling us: "You're not listening. I said, get out!!" This is called *the period of intensification*. It is just a little increase in anxiety, but very noticeable. During this brief period of intensification, we have an uneasy feeling that we are not approaching this problem correctly, and maybe our therapist doesn't know what they are talking about.

However, if you stay the course, usually in less than thirty minutes the anxiety will diminish and return to baseline. The brain will fire off the alarm, but the signal will weaken. On the next occasion we expose ourselves to the same cue (if close in time to the first exposure), the anxiety will spike up, but not as far as before. Again, if we remain exposed, the signal will weaken and eventually return to baseline. Each time we repeat the exposure, the power of the cue to elicit anxiety gets weaker and weaker until, finally, we no longer react to the cue.

For exposure to be effective, it must be systematic. The more close together in time that the exposures occur, the more effective the sessions are. If I have an elevator phobia but expose myself to elevators every few months when I have no choice, I will get little habituation. If I make it a point to ride an elevator once a month, the effect would be better, but not by much. Once a week would be better. Once a day is even better. The best would be to ride the elevator back-to-back eight to ten times in a row or until I experience very little reactivity, and then repeat the practice the next day. After a few days, I will probably no longer have an elevator phobia.

Anxiety and panic are analogous to a fire alarm that is not functioning properly. If its sensors are not calibrated correctly, the alarm
will go off when there is no fire. The noise of the alarm is loud, scary,
annoying, and very real. However, what is also very real is that there
is no fire. If I run out of the building thinking there is a fire, I leave
believing I narrowly escaped danger, and the next time I hear the fire
alarm, I will react even more readily. If I stay put for a few minutes, I
hear the announcement that it was a false alarm and everything is okay.

Right Action in these situations is to move toward the cue rather
than away. The more I move toward my conditioned fears systematically, the more room I have to feel peaceful rather than agitated toward
dangers that don't exist. However, our intuition and our hardwiring
tell us otherwise. We can choose Right Action to move toward a state
of well-being if we base our actions on Right Understanding of how
anxiety operates.

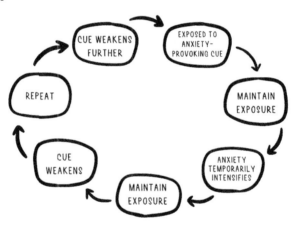

*Figure 13: Anxiety and Exposure Cycle*

Anxiety presses us to *do something*. When stewing about something
is making us anxious, we want to act, thinking that some action will
relieve our anxiety. Sometimes acting when we feel anxious might
resolve a problem or prevent it from becoming worse. However, on
other occasions, if we do nothing at all and gently hold our anxiety in
our awareness without feeling pressed to take action, the situation may
resolve on its own.

For example, when people suffer from an anxious attachment style,
they can become anxious when they do not hear from their partner.
*He hasn't texted me since yesterday morning . . . something must be wrong;*

*he may be mad about something . . . or blowing me off. I should talk to him or maybe confront him.* The anxiety is pressing for action. Often, if you wait for a bit, the situation will resolve itself. You may learn why he didn't text, and the reason is benign.

Imagine being in a pool with waves rising and falling. If you try to clear out the waves by swatting them down, all you do is create more waves. But if you allow yourself to be still and observe the waves, you notice that gradually they decrease until the water's surface is smooth. This is analogous to how our minds often work. Trying to make the anxiety go away is equivalent to slapping at the water and creating more disturbance on the surface. There is a time to act and a time not to act. Practice helps us to get good at telling the difference. There is an old Zen proverb along the lines of "Sitting quietly, doing nothing, spring comes, and the grass grows by itself."

We are hardwired and conditioned to feel like we must do something when anxious. I don't believe this proverb suggests we should only sit around doing nothing, especially if the house is on fire. The issue here is that the house is usually not on fire. We just react as though it is. Even when not in emergency mode, we often feel we must keep in motion, be productive, and keep doing something. Things often proceed just fine without us doing anything.

It is helpful here to bear in mind the wisdom of another Zen proverb: "The quieter you become, the more you are able to hear." We can often struggle with an exaggerated sense of self-importance. *Only I can handle this. If I don't make it happen, it won't happen.* However, imagine if you were gone—how would the world go on? Would the grass grow by itself?

## Anger

In Buddhism, anger is a negative emotion that can lead to negative actions and consequences. In this framework, we aim to understand the root cause of anger and healthily manage the feeling. The Buddha said: "Holding onto anger is like drinking poison and expecting the other person to die."

A Buddhist framework encourages us to look at the root cause of the anger. When we understand that anger is a mental state that arises due to certain conditions, such as desire, aversion, or failing to see things as they are, we can develop a deeper insight into anger, enabling us to be less reactive and to let go of it. Am I angry because of my desire to have things be my way? Am I suffering from aversion because my judging mind is causing me to feel ill will toward others, myself, or the current situation? Am I suffering from difficulty in seeing things as they are, such as not understanding the limits of my control and influence? Am I operating under the belief that my perspective is always the right one, and that anybody who views things differently is wrong?

I notice I feel angry. What is a skillful thing to do? A typical impulse is to vent my anger. However, if I typically rely on venting to cope with anger, I may feel better in the short run, but over time I might notice that it takes less and less provocation to make me angry.

Studies have found that high anger in response to stress in young men is associated with an increased risk of premature cardiovascular disease, particularly myocardial infarction (Chang et al., 2002) and an increased risk of death in those already diagnosed with cardiovascular disease (Verrier & Mittleman, 1996; Siegman, 1993). Venting anger does not appear to be such a good idea.

So, if venting is not a good idea, how about suppression? If we try to ignore our anger, we are likely to express it in harmful ways like passive-aggressive behavior, or it could even transform into depression. Sometimes we can get into a destructive cycle where we vent anger and get bad or unsatisfactory results. So on the next several occasions, we suppress our anger but nurture negative thoughts. The anger builds to where we can no longer suppress it, and then we explode. When we've cooled down, we feel bad, and then the cycle repeats itself. In the Buddhist framework, this is a manifestation of the poison of aversion. I don't like feeling angry, so I fight with it and suppress it.

This dilemma of venting vs. suppressing comes from thinking of anger as "steam." If you vent it, someone may get burned. If you don't vent it, the "pressure" builds up, and you have no choice but to vent. Another frame is to ask ourselves, *Why is there steam in the pot in the first place? What about the stove is creating conditions favorable for steam?*

### What Causes Anger?

I have found it very useful to view anger as usually resulting from one of two conditions:

- Misdirected control
- An unexpressed unmet need

The first and more typical cause is *misdirected control*. This is an effort to control the wrong thing. We experience anger when we try to control something that, in reality, we have no control over. The vast universe of things we have no control over includes all the things beyond the ends of our fingertips. Next time you feel angry, look at the end of your fingertips. Consider everything that is beyond the tips of your finger. All of those things are comprise the universe of things over which you have no control.

We don't control other people, how they act, their choices, or how they think. We don't control "out there." We don't control things that have already happened. We don't control events that unfold unfairly.

A good occasion to practice this concept is the next time you are stuck in traffic and feeling angry or frustrated. It is not the traffic making the anger. Your mind wants to control the traffic, when actually you have no control over it. You will arrive when you arrive based on the conditions. The only question is will you arrive late and angry or merely late? This is a good time to look at your fingertips and remind yourself where your control stops.

*Well, I have control over my young children, don't I?* No, you have responsibility *for* your children, but no control. If a two-year-old has the mind to throw a tantrum in the grocery store, they will. You have no control over that, only how you react to that as a parent.

It is hard for some individuals to come to terms with the reality of the limits of our control. There is comfort in living in the delusion that we move the pieces of our life around and the universe bends to our will. However, this sets us up to experience either anger or helplessness. It is empowering to understand that I only have control over myself, because now I will only expend energy on attempting to control the single thing over which I actually do have control.

Recognizing the limits of one's control is not the same as being passive. I still may try to influence the situation. But I will proceed without anger if I have clarity regarding what I actually have control over. Ironically, I can often be more influential in a situation by only controlling myself. For example, if I accept the bumper-to-bumper traffic and nurture healthy thoughts, I will eventually arrive at my destination free from self-created stress and likely in a pleasant mood. This differs greatly from swearing, pressing my horn, or weaving in and out recklessly, and arriving in a foul mood.

About eighty percent of the time, anger results from misdirected control. Roughly the other twenty percent of the time, we experience anger when we have *an unexpressed unmet need*. We get angry at someone for not addressing the need we failed to tell them about. We might adopt the dysfunctional relationship belief of *mind reading is expected*. This belief is the idea that if I have to tell someone my needs, they are diminishes somehow. The dysfunctional thought is *I shouldn't have to tell you my needs. If you loved me, you would just know.* Or another version: *Great. You are only doing that because I asked you to*, as if that's a bad thing.

Anger and anxiety have a similar physiological footprint of a heightened level of arousal. The first step in dealing with anger is to address automatic physiological arousal. Remember that you get good at what you practice. If you have practiced anger for some time, you have become good at it. You have cultivated neural circuits in your brain that are on standby and ready to react angrily whenever threatened. The "pause" between the trigger and the reaction is very brief. By practicing downregulating the arousal that goes with anger, you can increase the pause between trigger and reaction (See "Breathing Techniques to Calm Overarousal" later in this chapter).

### Forgiveness

We need to understand that the wish of ill-will rarely harms the difficult person. It harms us by being attached to our hurt and our suffering. Instead, we can practice shifting focus.

Usually, when someone hurts us, our initial reflex is to think, *Isn't it awful being me and suffering this person?* In the practice of shifting focus, instead of entangling ourselves with our own suffering, we focus on the other person's suffering. *Would I want to be that person? Of course not!* Why? If we think deeply beyond our reactive reflex, we realize that the other party suffers by being who they are. They may suffer from anger, ignorance, arrogance, and lack of empathy. They suffer from various things that make them difficult or hurtful.Part of practicing loving-kindness is having a practice of forgiveness. When we practice forgiving, we let go of negative feelings or any desire for punishment, retribution, or compensation. The word itself contains the meaning "to give away." I like the idea of *I forgive you. I give back to you what was yours before (your bad act). It is up to you to make your peace with it (or not). I choose to carry it no longer.* When I hold on to hurt or anger, it is like carrying the other person's karma for them. When I forgive, I let them carry their own karma.

A few things can impede practicing forgiveness. First, we get caught if we view forgiveness as a gift we give the other person. There is an old saying: "Forgive others not because they deserve it, but because you deserve peace." When we view forgiveness as something we give the other person, we hesitate, getting caught up in measuring whether they are worthy. Second, we might think we somehow have to minimize the bad act. Sometimes we do this for casual events: "It's no big deal. Don't give it another thought." What about when the hurt is not superficial? It is essential to understand that it is not necessary to minimize the hurt to practice forgiveness.

Third, forgiveness is not like a light switch that you turn on or off. It is more like a state of mind that that you practice. Sometimes we let go, and then grab on to the hurt again and wish for retribution. The practice is to keep letting go. Finally, I have noticed that people struggle with forgiveness when they conflate it with vulnerability. *If I forgive this person, I must be vulnerable again, and they might hurt me. If I hang onto my anger, they cannot hurt me.* You can forgive someone while understanding that deciding whether to be vulnerable is a separate matter.

### The 3 Rs: The Foundation for Vulnerability
If someone hurts me, I practice forgiveness for my sake. By practicing forgiveness, I work on cultivating a mindset that is peaceful instead of filled with hurt and resentment.

Being vulnerable is a different consideration. I may forgive you, but being emotionally vulnerable with you is an entirely different thing. I have found the concept of the "3Rs" to be helpful in this context. If someone hurts you, they are likely to repeat that behavior unless they work the 3Rs: *recognition, remorse, and repair.*

*Recognition* refers to the other's party's understanding of how their actions affected you. This is beyond the obvious. Do they understand the effects in some detail? How did the act jeopardize your trust, your view of the world, and your sense of self? Next, having recognized the effects of their actions, do they exhibit indications of *remorse*? Not merely feeling bad because you are angry with them, but does their regret or guilt arise from compassion for how you are affected? Do they feel remorse because they fully recognize the consequences of their actions? Finally, do they make *repair*? Repair entails making efforts to mitigate the harm already caused and taking appropriate steps to ensure it will not happen again.

The party needs to exhibit all 3 Rs. If someone doesn't even recognize how their actions impacted you, they will probably repeat the act. If they realize the impact but don't care, they will probably hurt you again. If they recognize the hurt and genuinely feel remorse, but don't take steps to mitigate harm or prevent reoccurrence, you are at risk of being hurt again.

Vulnerability, like forgiveness, is not an all-or-nothing process. It is a matter of degree. You can use the framework of the 3Rs to help calibrate how vulnerable to be. If the person exhibits some degree of all three, then you can risk being a little vulnerable. If the person does solid, genuine work on all three, then you can allow yourself to be more vulnerable. If there is a complete absence of the 3Rs, then it is probably unwise to allow yourself to be vulnerable with that person.

## Insomnia

Restful sleep is essential for cultivating a peaceful mind. Unfortunately, if our mind is not peaceful, the first thing that gets out of balance is our sleep. For this reason, *insomnia*—defined as difficulty falling asleep or staying asleep, or waking up too early—is very common when struggling with stress or mental health issues. Taking Right Action with respect to our sleep is a key aspect to the Eightfold Path.

Insomnia can be acute (short term) or chronic (long term). According to the American Academy of Sleep Medicine, approximately thirty percent of adults have symptoms of insomnia, with about ten percent experiencing chronic insomnia. Other estimates suggest that up to fifty percent of adults experience occasional insomnia. Insomnia can be a symptom of an underlying medical or psychiatric condition, so it's important to consult with an appropriate professional if you are experiencing persistent sleep difficulties. As with other aspects of Right Action, in the case of insomnia, Right Action can be counterintuitive.

*Sleep hygiene* is a set of habits and practices that can help to promote good-quality sleep. Good sleep hygiene can correct many issues with insomnia without the use of medication.

### Rule #1 of Sleep Hygiene

"Never have insomnia in bed." When I share this suggestion with folks, they often are puzzled, thinking, *Well, where else would I have it?* When you experience the discomfort of insomnia in your bed, the anxiety associated with insomnia becomes stimulus-bound with the bed and other cues in the bedroom. The bedroom itself *cues* insomnia.

Instead of tossing and turning in bed, try the following. If you have not fallen asleep within fifteen to twenty minutes, get out of bed, go to another room, and engage in a quiet activity. Only return to bed when you feel drowsy. Again, if you do not fall asleep within fifteen to twenty minutes, get back out of bed and repeat the process above. Do this as often as necessary throughout the night. Do NOT try to make yourself sleep. Sleep is a passive process; the harder you try to sleep, the more difficult it is to fall asleep.

## Other sleep hygiene practices

* Establish a consistent wake time. If you usually get up at 7 a.m. when not experiencing insomnia, then get up at this time regardless of how bad the night before was. The biggest mistake in coping with insomnia is trying to catch up on sleep lost the night before. Sleeping during the day worsens the problem. When you have a very long nap in the middle of what should be your wake cycle it disrupts your circadian rhythm. Your body's circadian rhythm, or "body clock," works like a timer running backwards. A long nap "resets" the clock and the brain gets a little confused about what "body time" it is. It is also crucial to expose yourself to sunlight or other bright light as soon as possible after waking. This gives your brain a clear signal that the daytime part of the cycle has begun, which will then make you more receptive to sleep as the clock ticks down.

- Remain awake for a complete daytime cycle. Avoid napping unless you are unable to stay awake. Only indulge in a nap when your sleep cycle is stable.
- Avoid caffeine in coffee, tea, sodas, and other foods. Avoid herbal supplements that have stimulant properties. If your caffeine intake is high, gradually reduce it until you are entirely off caffeine. Abrupt cessation of caffeine can cause headaches and fatigue.
- If you tend to think a lot about problems around bedtime, try writing your thoughts and feelings in a journal before attempting to sleep. This practice leads many people to experience a decrease in ruminative thinking. If you have many tasks on your plate, develop a ritual early in the evening to review your to-do list, adding and checking items off. When you journal or cull your to-do list, rumination diminishes. It's as if your mind is satisfied that there is a "hard copy" and stops recycling the thoughts.
- Establish a bedtime routine. If you ask people what their nighttime ritual is, people who sleep well will usually say something like: "After supper, I go for a walk, close out my computer, and then take a warm bath. I put the coffee on for the morning

and take the dog outside one last time. My spouse and I get in bed and read, then fall asleep." The answer will be the same five or six things, usually done in the same order almost every night. This routine performed in a predictable order serves as a cue to the brain that the day is ending and sleep is approaching. On the other hand, if I do a bunch of random things and then jump into bed, my brain is not prepared to receive sleep.

At least one to two hours before retiring for the night, begin a regular routine that is conducive to sleep. Avoid complicated tasks or vigorous exercise in this interval before bedtime. Ask yourself if your activities during this interval help with "winding down" from the day. Try taking a warm bath or listening to soft music. Avoid stimulating activities. Make sure the lighting is low. Bright lights suppress your brain's production of melatonin, a brain chemical involved in sleep initiation. Avoid screen time on electronic devices.

- Get aerobic exercise. A little moderate aerobic activity, such as a relaxed walk, in the late afternoon or early evening goes a long way toward relieving physical and mental stress and contributes to being prepared for sleep.
- Avoid alcohol. It may sedate you for the night's first half, but the second half can be fraught with increased awakenings and light sleep. If you struggle with insomnia in the middle of the night, alcohol can often be a factor.
- Don't try too hard. The harder you try, the more awake you'll become. Nothing will chase the sandman away faster than the thought: *Oh no, I hope I'm not going to have insomnia.*

Try to follow the suggestions above faithfully for ten to fourteen days. If the problem persists, you may be experiencing an issue more complicated than simple insomnia and may want to consult a psychologist. Clinical depression, anxiety disorder, and other mental health problems can manifest with sleep disturbance. If the underlying cause is correctly diagnosed and treated, the insomnia will resolve.

Prescription sleep medications can be effective for helping people fall asleep and stay asleep, but they come with potential risks and side effects, such as drowsiness, impaired cognitive function, and dependency. In addition, many prescription sleep medications are only intended for short-term use, and they often result in rebound insomnia when discontinued. In contrast, good sleep hygiene practices are generally considered safe and without side effects. It may take some effort to establish a consistent sleep routine and make the necessary lifestyle changes to improve sleep quality, but consider the payoff in long-term health and well-being.

If you would prefer to stay away from prescription sleep medications, there is some evidence that zinc, magnesium, and melatonin are effective interventions for simple insomnia. One study of older adults found that a combination of magnesium and melatonin significantly improved sleep quality and duration (Abbasi et al., 2012).

## Breathing Techniques to Calm Overarousal

One thing that anxiety, depression, anger, and insomnia can have in common is *overarousal*. Overarousal is when we get stuck in a stress response. The arousal stays high like a stuck gas pedal. An approach that helps to reduce overarousal is regulation of the breath. Often referred to as *paced breathing* (Stancák et al., 1993), these breathing techniques are based on slowing the frequency of breath cycles per minute. Paced breathing has been found to evoke relaxation and well-being (Jerath et al., 2015), while fast breathing has been linked to anxiety and stress (Homma & Masaoka, 2008; Zaccaro, 2017). If you imagine yourself sitting in a comfortable chair outside, relaxing and watching the sunset, you will notice your breathing is naturally slow and low in the abdomen. If you imagine hiding behind a tree from a bad guy trying to hurt you, you will notice your breathing is rapid, shallow, and high in the chest.

### 2-10 Breathing

To downregulate the overarousal associated with negative feelings, we can slow our breathing. Here's how.

1. Sit comfortably where you won't be disturbed. Set a timer for ten minutes. Then pick a spot across the room on which to fix your gaze.
2. Breathe from your diaphragm. To check if you are doing this, place your hand on your lower abdomen. When you breathe in, you should feel your tummy expand outward, then deflate when you exhale. Your chest and shoulders should not move as much.
3. Next, make the exhalation about five times longer than the inhalation. For example, aim to breathe in for a count of two, then exhale for a count of ten. (One count = approximately one second.)
4. Finally, slow your respiration rate to about five cycles per minute. The math works out like this: (inhale for two seconds + exhale for ten seconds) twelve seconds × five rounds = sixty seconds,

meaning that in one minute we can do roughly five cycles of paced breathing.

5. Continue with the cycles of breath, keeping your gaze on your chosen point, until you are relaxed or the timer sounds.

It can feel awkward at first if you run out of air at about count five on the exhalation and cannot make it to ten. Think of it as letting air out of a balloon in a slow and a controlled fashion. There is also no problem with exhaling longer than a ten count as long as you are not straining.

It is essential to *practice* this technique. It will work somewhat if you only do it when you're upset. However, it will work many times better if you have been practicing it regularly. With practice, the neural pathways become easier to access, especially when you need them. Practice this breathing pattern once or twice (or more) daily. After ten minutes or so of breathing in this manner, you should experience a much lower level of arousal than when you started. You should also find that over time it does not take ten minutes to achieve a relaxed state, but only a few breaths.

### Let Go Breathing

We have discussed the importance of understanding the connection between attachment and suffering. A brief exercise that can serve as a reminder about this connection is to draw in a full breath and hold it—don't exhale. Here's how:

1. Hold your breath. Stay attached to it. Stubbornly refuse to let go.
2. Eventually, reality intrudes and you must "let go." Exhale fully.
3. Now you feel a sense of relief. This is letting go.

Notice that at times when you feel resistant to a situation, you feel tight and are subtly holding your breath. Then notice that if you change your mind and stop resisting the situation, you might let out a sigh—letting go of the breath as you let go of your resistance to the situation.

## Repeatedly in the *Problem State*

Dialectical behavior therapy (DBT) is a more specific form of CBT that focuses on helping people with extreme emotional reactions interact with their environment in a less emotional, healthier way. DBT relies heavily on mindfulness skills used in Buddhism and Zen practices. DBT teaches patients to use specific mindfulness techniques to learn to live with pain in the world and accept how things are instead of suffering by trying to change them.

DBT has been empirically validated for a variety of populations and issues, including substance use disorders, suicide attempts, PTSD, self-harm, symptoms of depression and anxiety, and eating disorders (Vaughn, 2021).

This therapy was originally developed in the late 1970s by Marsha Linehan. Through careful examination and trial and error, she found an approach that balanced accountability with support. Linehan is now a Zen master. During her earlier training, she found that many of the principles she was learning in Zen and in her meditation were applicable to the populations she worked with as a psychologist, and mindfulness was one of them.

In a Buddhist framework, part of the practice is to be mindful of conditions that create negative mental states. Marsha Linehan developed a tool for understanding conditions that give rise to a *problem state*, which in this context refers to any behavioral pattern that occurs repeatedly, even though it may be regretted. For example, I may drink too much. The next day I am hung over and vow that I'm never going to do that again. Yet, the next happy hour I drink too much again, feel bad, make the same vow . . . rinse and repeat.

The basic idea of this behavior analysis tool is that problem states do not suddenly occur for no reason. They arise out of conditions, as do all things. These conditions usually involve a chain of states that, if left unchecked, eventually lead to the problem state. Understanding our behavioral chain allows us to adopt Right Action and to keep our actions from involving self-harm or harm to others.

The first link in the chain is *vulnerability*. This state is basically when we feel out of sorts emotionally, and it is usually not a result of just one thing. More often, it is an accumulation of events, and then at a particular juncture, there is a tipping point where we are now in a vulnerable state. The behavioral chain occurs over the course of a unit of time, such as a day, or more extended periods, like a week or a month.

For example, I might have slept poorly last night. That is troublesome, but I'm still okay. Maybe I also am coming down with a cold. Still OK. Then I argue with my spouse, but I am still mostly OK. Then I have a flat tire on the way to work, and when I arrive at work, I get yelled at by my boss. I have reached the tipping point, and now I feel vulnerable and out of sorts.

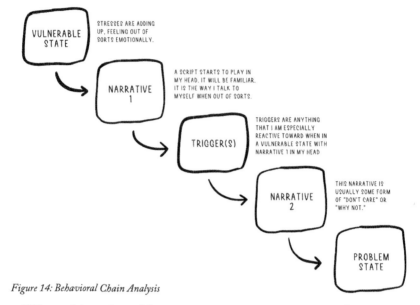

STRESSES ARE ADDING
UP, FEELING OUT OF
SORTS EMOTIONALLY.

VULNERABLE
STATE

A SCRIPT STARTS TO PLAY IN
MY HEAD. IT WILL BE FAMILIAR.
IT IS THE WAY I TALK TO
MYSELF WHEN OUT OF SORTS.

NARRATIVE
1

TRIGGERS ARE ANYTHING
THAT I AM ESPECIALLY
REACTIVE TOWARD WHEN IN
A VULNERABLE STATE WITH
NARRATIVE 1 IN MY HEAD

TRIGGER(S)

THIS NARRATIVE IS
USUALLY SOME FORM
OF "DON'T CARE" OR
"WHY NOT."

NARRATIVE
2

PROBLEM
STATE

*Figure 14: Behavioral Chain Analysis*

When this vulnerable state occurs, we may notice that a *narrative* plays in our head. This narrative is usually very personal and will often feel familiar. It is the familiar way we grumble internally when feeling emotionally vulnerable. There is an infinite number of variations, but common narratives might have a theme like *Woe is me, No one appreciates/understands me, Why me? The world is going to hell,* and so on. When in a vulnerable state, out of habit we usually gravitate toward a familiar narrative.

Once we are vulnerable and the narrative is playing in our head, we are much more reactive to *triggers*. A trigger is anything we are reactive toward that speeds up our advancement toward the problem state. Triggers are as varied as the people exposed to them. For example, your dysfunctional family may trigger you by inviting you out to eat Mexican food when you have an eating disorder. Or it might be your friend asking you to go have a beer, "code" for "let's go out and get hammered." Or it might be your partner gaslighting you about an event you know did not happen the way he claims. It could be not being chosen for the new position at work.

Once we are triggered, what often happens next is that the narrative now shifts to one along the lines of *Why not? Who cares? I deserve X. The heck with it, I'm just going to do . . .* Once this narrative plays in our head, we are very close to entering the problem state. The problem state is usually some self-defeating or self-harming behavior that we have often done and each time vowed never to do again, yet here we find ourselves in the same place again.

As we pass through each link in the chain, we build up more and more behavioral momentum. It gets harder and harder to change direction. However, at each link, we can develop "off-ramps" to take us off the behavioral chain.

For each off-ramp, you must have a written plan you can refer to. It is important to develop these plans not when you are in crisis but when you feel centered. We don't have access to our creative selves when stressed out emotionally. Writing helps in recognizing the particular link in the chain, and then the corresponding antidote or off-ramp.

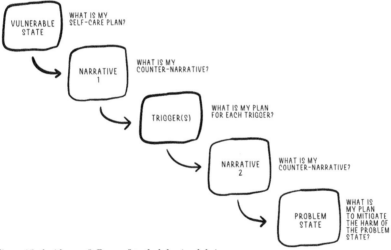

*Figure 15: Antidotes or "off-ramps" to the behavioral chain.*

*Vulnerability.* Remember that vulnerability is a state where you feel stressed and emotionally out of sorts. The antidotes for this state will usually entail self-care. Self-care is a personal matter. Everyone's approach will be different. Self-care refers to activities that you use to decompress and recharge emotionally. If you ignore your self-care, stress will accumulate and manifest adverse effects. If the vulnerability is not addressed, you will probably move on to the next link in the chain.

It is essential to be aware of the stress–self-care paradox. I've been visiting with people about stress for a long time. Some people seldom engage in self-care and must learn how to implement these things from scratch. Others will have a self-care routine they happily engage in when their stress levels are in the green zone, but when their stress redlines, self-care is often the first to go. It is better to be sure and engage is self-care when the stress levels rise: *I've had a bad day. I need a workout, or a hot bath, or to go to bed early.*

Use your calendar to allot time for self-care. One study on the habits of successful people found that they regularly scheduled self-care items like going to the gym or doing a hobby, just as they would business meetings or appointments with a doctor. We often approach self-care items as something we do only if the time is free. If that is your approach, you will often find that other things routinely push out self-care. Make it a priority to bring a better you to the party.

*Narrative 1.* Remember, Narrative 1 plays in your head when you feel emotionally out of sorts. This narrative usually contains unskillful thoughts that sustain or magnify the vulnerable state. Once you have reflected on your narrative and written it down, the task is to construct a counter-narrative. One way to construct a counter-narrative is to reframe any cognitive distortions embedded in the narrative (see chapter 4, Right Thought). Another way to construct a counter-narrative is to think of a worldview you would like to aspire to and then try to put it into words. If you have inspirational quotes or sayings that reflect your desired worldview, you can include them in a new narrative. Write the counter-narrative and put it where you can easily access it when you need it.

*Triggers.* Suppose you know that when you are entangled in the behavioral chain, certain things trigger you. It is crucial to have a plan to avoid the trigger altogether or, if confronted with it, to mitigate its effect. If I know I am out of sorts, I might decline Joe's invitation to go have a few beers. I might avoid family for now. I might not expose myself to cable news or social media. If I can't avoid Joe or family, do I have a script prepared to help me decline an invitation or clarify a boundary?

*Narrative 2.* The approach for Narrative 2 is very similar to that for Narrative 1. The work is to first put into writing Narrative 2. Remember, this is usually some form of *don't care, why not, I deserve*, and so forth. The goal is to write up a counter-narrative. Do you really not care? Instead, what do you care about? Answer the question "Why not?" What is likely to happen if you enter the problem state?

*Problem State.* Now you can develop a plan to mitigate the harmful effects of the problem state. For example, if I go out with Joe and get hammered, what is my plan? Maybe get an Uber instead of driving intoxicated? What is my plan to reset, rather than feel like I've gone back to square one? When developing the plan for the problem state, the mindset is to acknowledge that you've fallen into the hole, and but there's no need to dig it deeper. Your plan will stop you from tossing more dirt over the side of the hole.

Remember, the key notion of this journey is to pay attention to conditions that give rise to suffering. Suffering usually doesn't just visit us randomly. It incrementally sneaks up on us. That's why it's important to pay attention and be mindful. You never know what may be sneaking up on you!

## The Path Forward . . .

The Eightfold Path has been built on the foundation of the wisdom of seeing things as they are and cultivating thoughts that reflect this understanding. Standing firmly on this base of wisdom, we then conduct ourselves ethically in our speech and actions with the aim to reduce suffering in ourselves and others. We explored examples of how our actions can sometimes make things worse and that the more skillful path is sometimes counterintuitive. Both Buddhist and CBT frameworks stress the importance of paying attention to patterns in our thinking that lead to suffering or problem states, and to the conditions that give rise to these states.

Take a moment to ask yourself what concept(s) in this chapter offered a perspective you had not considered before. Going forward what actions might you practice to support a feeling of well-being in yourself and others? Is there a specific behavior you have that you notice contributes to your stress? Can you identify the conditions that lead to this behavior?

In the next chapter, we will explore how we practice the Path while in the world of work. The way in which we earn a livelihood provides many opportunities to practice skillfully. It can also create conditions that can undermine our practice.

# 7

# RIGHT LIVELIHOOD

*"Right livelihood is the art of finding fulfillment in work that uplifts ourselves and others, where our vocation becomes a source of joy, meaning, and service to the world."*

*– Jack Kornfield*

# Buddhism and Right Livelihood

Right Livelihood refers to making a living in a way that avoids harm to yourself and others and is ethically positive. Remember, each of the practices of the Eightfold Path relates to and reinforces each of the others. If I have a good practice going for seven out of the eight but work as a hitman or drug dealer, my choice of livelihood will probably undermine my overall practice.

Right Livelihood entails being mindful of how work affects your heart and mind. Is it a support or a hindrance? Does my work increase my happiness and wisdom or relieve suffering in myself and others? Does it facilitate a calm mind?

In general, Right Livelihood means avoiding occupations that produce harm. There is no discouragement of making profits or accumulating wealth. It just must be done legally, peacefully, without violence, and honestly, without deceit. It must not harm others. It is easy to see how some occupations might not be Right Livelihood. An assassin and a drug dealer would not meet the criteria of avoiding harm to others. However, as with many ethical considerations, things are not always cut and dried. For example, imagine I work as a manager. I conduct myself ethically, treat my colleagues and staff kindly, and work diligently. However, I work for a company that sells a product that harms people. I would have to determine whether the work supports or undermines my practice.

How we earn our living rarely occurs in a vacuum. We have customers, coworkers, supervisors, and the public with whom we interact. When we engage in work, we are not an isolated entity unto ourselves but interdependent within a larger context. We therefore have many opportunities to practice Right Understanding, Right Thought, Right Action, and Right Speech daily in our working lives.

# CBT and Right Livelihood

## Work-Life Balance

An essential part of Right Livelihood is finding a balance between your work and non-work life. A necessary first step in developing a good work-life balance involves setting clear boundaries separating work from the rest of life. We are less stressed when we have clear boundaries around our work. You must have a clear distinction that indicates your work is now done and you are starting nonwork life.

This clear distinction is often difficult to establish for people who run a business out of their home. There is always the temptation to do "one more thing," and there is a feeling of never really being off. More and more people have been working remotely during and since the pandemic of 2020, and for many this has blurred the work-life boundaries.

Another problem is that we often receive work-related electronic communications after hours. This doesn't have to be a problem. It depends on how much it disturbs your focus. When the boundaries between work and nonwork are fuzzy, we will often think about home when at work and think about work when we are home.

The Harvard Longitudinal Study on Adult Development, also known as the Grant Study,[2] is one of the longest-running studies of human development (Vaillant, 2012). It began in 1938 and has followed the lives of 268 male Harvard undergraduates for over eighty years, studying their physical and mental health, career trajectories, relationships, and overall well-being. The study has expanded several times to now include over 1800 participants across the generations.

One of the study's main findings is that close relationships are crucial to happiness and well-being. The study found that people who were more socially connected to family, friends, and community were happier, healthier, and lived longer than those who were more isolated. This finding held across the lifespan, from adolescence to old age. Another key result is that having a sense of purpose in life is vital for happiness and well-being. The study found that people with a clear sense of direction and meaning in life and who pursued personally meaningful goals were happier and more fulfilled than those without. These results suggest that we can improve our happiness by nurturing close relationships, finding purpose, and cultivating resilience in adversity.

It is essential to be mindful of how work affects these aspects of happiness. I might have work that brings positive relationships that

2    *This book summarizes the findings from the Grant Study, as well as the more recent studies that have built upon its work. It provides a detailed account of the study's design, methods, and key findings, and includes many personal stories and insights from the participants themselves. It also discusses the implications of the study's findings for our understanding of human development and well-being. There are many other articles and publications based on the Grant Study that can be found through a search of academic databases or by visiting the Harvard Study of Adult Development website.*

support my journey. I might have work that takes my time away from my close relationships, like family and friends. I might have a job that feels purposeful or one that sucks the life out of me.

## Toxic Work Environments

You might do work that does not cause harm to others and is ethically positive, but the work environment itself might be toxic. This situation can result from abusive coworkers, a manager who is often offensive and manipulative, or systemic factors such as a chronically understaffed workgroup and upper-level management making financial decisions that do not consider staff well-being. Toxic environments like this create unnecessary suffering.

As with a toxic interpersonal relationship, in a toxic work environment we have four main response choices: change, accept, leave, or limbo.

*Change.* We can ask ourselves: "What in this situation can I change?" Maybe I can work on confronting abusive behavior. If I am criticized, I may try to be less defensive. Can I change how I react to situations in my work environment? Is there anything I can do differently about interacting with other parties at work? Can I change how I allow the situation to affect me?

*Accept.* Sometimes you can try every which way to make healthy changes, but nothing works. The toxic nature of the situation persists. The next thing to ask yourself is "Can I work at acceptance?" Often things are stressful because we don't accept things as they are. I may have a boss or coworker who behaves badly. Is the problem the behavior or my difficulty in accepting the behavior?

Sometimes people confuse acceptance with preference. Acceptance does not mean you approve of the situation, condone destructive behavior, or prefer things this way. Acceptance means aligning with the reality of the situation. If the boss usually behaves in a selfish and rude manner, acceptance helps me not to be shocked and amazed every time they act in character. We can healthily work on acceptance.

*Leave.* If things are not changing and I cannot accept how things are, I might consider leaving. I could ask for a transfer to another workgroup or find another job that is not toxic. One effect of stress, particularly the kind that comes from an unhealthy situation, is tunnel vision—a narrow view that makes it hard to explore options. That can lead to a feeling of being trapped, as if there are no viable options, but that is rarely the case. I might feel that there are no options because I feel trapped by all the givens I take for granted. For example, I must live in a half-million-dollar house, drive expensive cars, and go on expensive vacations. I take this lifestyle as fixed and fret about maintaining it, rather than considering that it might be best for me to leave and cultivate a different situation. We can then work on leaving thoughtfully and healthily.

*Limbo.* The last approach is limbo. Limbo is when things are not changing, I cannot accept things as they are, and I am not leaving the situation. Limbo is the only one that we cannot do healthily. Limbo feels like perpetual stress over the same things over and over again.

### The Illusion of Everything Is the Most Important

A workgroup that is understaffed creates some toxic situations. Staff departures have led to fewer people doing the same volume of work. Of course, the remaining staff are not being paid two salaries despite doing the work of two people. This situation, unfortunately, is common. Higher-level management sometimes makes decisions that do not consider staff well-being.

In this situation, eventually it will be the case that you have more things on your to-do list than can reasonably be completed in a workday. A good manager will recognize the task overload and help you prioritize to give attention to the most important tasks and let the least important ones slide a bit, understanding that under the circumstances not everything will get done.

However, sometimes managers are stressed out by their managers or are just poor managers. When you ask them what you should prioritize, you will receive some version of "It's all important. Just get it done." If you persist and ask, "Yes, but what is the most important?" you will receive no clear direction.

We can think of a typical to-do list as having A, B, and C tasks. "A" tasks are the most important ones. They are the ones that reflect the central functioning of the position. They are mission-critical and will usually have harmful consequences if not completed. "B" tasks are important but only support mission-critical tasks. "C" tasks are part of the job and are unimportant, but they can sometimes be urgent. The list may shuffle as time passes, due dates approach, and so on. When we prioritize a list of tasks, at the very top of the list is A1, the most important of all the tasks.

Imagine a situation where the work is on task overload, and your manager asks you to do one more thing. You were already doing the other thing she asked you to do. Which of the two should be the A1 task? If she is a poor manager, you will get some version of "It's all important. Just get it done." I like to refer to this as "the illusion of multiple A1 tasks." It is an illusion because you cannot have two things that are the most. You can only have one thing that is the most. Under these circumstances, you must prioritize using your best judgment and allow the chips to fall where they may. You will not get everything done, but you will have completed the most important things. If the work environment is out of touch with reality and expects everything to be of equal importance and that everything must be done, then it might be healthier to find work that is more aligned with reality.

If you cannot remove yourself from a toxic work environment, then the practice is to mitigate the negative effects of stress until conditions change. General self-care is essential here, especially meditation practice and exercise (see chapter 10). It is critical to have some stress-offsetting strategies. Otherwise, the toxic effects of stress will accumulate and affect your well-being, physical health, and close relationships.

## Relationship between Money and Happiness

Research has shown a correlation between money and happiness, but it is not a direct, consistent one. Generally, people with enough money to meet their basic needs such as a place to live, food, and healthcare, are happier than those without. However, once those basic needs are met, additional money does not significantly impact happiness.

Kahneman and Deaton (2020) found that emotional well-being increased with each dollar added to income up to about seventy-five thousand dollars.[3] After that, each extra dollar added to the salary provided a rapidly diminishing happiness return. This led researchers to study the idea that people seem to adapt to wealth quickly. You buy a new car or toy. The initial excitement wears off, and a month or two later, you are used to it.

Whatever the magic number is, other factors account for happiness beyond that number. One of these is discretionary time. Studies of the relationship between individuals' discretionary time and subjective well-being show that, whereas having too little time is indeed linked

---

3    *Subjects were U.S. citizens. The dollar amount would likely vary greatly among different countries.*

to lower subjective well-being caused by stress, having more time does not continually translate to greater subjective well-being. Having an abundance of discretionary time is sometimes even linked to lower subjective well-being because of a lack of productivity or purpose, but that effect is reduced when the discretionary time is spent on productive activities. The "ideal" range was two to five hours per day. Less than two hours was associated with a decline in well-being, as was more than five hours (Sharif, 2021). So, making more money beyond basic needs at the expense of discretionary time may actually lead to a decrease in happiness.

Financial abundance can also bring problems, such as stress, anxiety, and social isolation. Material possessions and wealth can temporarily create happiness, but it doesn't last long. A sense of purpose, meaningful relationships, and a fulfilling life are critical factors for happiness and well-being. Studies show that people who enjoy a windfall by winning a lottery get a temporary bump in happiness that fades quickly to pre-win baseline levels. Some winners even become less happy after the windfall. They buy costly items, such as a second house or a boat, and then find that they have less discretionary time because they are taking care of all of their new "stuff." Some people become less happy because of the negative impact of their suddenly increased wealth on existing relationships.

In summary, more money can bring more happiness, but only up to a certain point. Beyond that, other factors, such as personal relationships, mental and physical health, and a sense of purpose, impact happiness more. If you make a great deal of money, but the stress of doing so compromises your health and close relationships, you may not achieve the happiness you are hoping for.

Let's imagine a not-uncommon scenario. I already make a pretty good living—my basic needs are met, and my family has two cars, health insurance, money for vacations, and solid savings. I get offered a new job with a twenty-thousand-dollar bump in salary. Unfortunately, the job is on the other side of town with a one-hour commute. The corporate culture encourages working long hours.

I may find that I am happy I am successful in my career (life satisfaction), but I do not enjoy emotional well-being in my day-to-day life. I have more money, but it is not significantly impacting my lifestyle. The extra hours and the commute have diminished discretionary time that I might spend with friends and family, exercising, or pursuing a hobby. Thus we can see that having neither too little nor too much discretionary time can be another example of the Middle Way in a Buddhist framework.

## Retirement

At some point in most people's lives, their means of earning a livelihood changes. They may be fortunate to have saved and invested well and can now support their lifestyle without exchanging their time and labor (mental or physical) for money. We call this retirement. What does the practice of Right Livelihood look like during this period of life?

Interestingly, people consider money and time differently when planning for retirement. Often people will plan financially for retirement many years in advance. They create detailed budgets. How they will spend their money is often laid out very carefully.

But they often do not give the same careful consideration to how they will spend their time, even though time and money are both finite resources. I have noticed that this lack of consideration often leads to subtle unhappiness for people after retirement. They may plan to get certain projects around the house finally completed or take the long-desired vacation, but after a year or so, the vacation is done, and so are the projects. Now what?

Just like during our working years, it is crucial to have a purpose. What is my "work" after I retire? When I wake up in the morning, why do I get out of bed? I often think about the word purpose. We have the phrase "on purpose," which implies that I mean to do something purposefully instead of approaching it accidentally. It implies intentionality.

*Ikigai* is a Japanese word roughly translated as "reason for living, purpose in life, or raison d'être." Our ikigai is the reason we get up in the morning. "One surprising thing you notice, living in Japan, is how active people remain after they retire. Many Japanese people never really retire—they keep doing what they love for as long as their health allows" (Garcia, 2017, p. 9). There are various places in the world called "blue zones," where there are unusual concentrations of people who live to extreme old age. One of these blue zones in is Okinawa. One common factor among the centenarians there is a sense of ikigai.

## The Path Forward . . .

The Path presents many opportunities to practice in the context of how we earn a living. The foundation of wisdom gained from Right

Understanding and Right Thought can apply to how we deal with co-workers, supervisors, clients, or the public. If we are mindful, we can notice the ways our work supports our journey healthily or undermines it.

So far there is quite a bit to pay attention to on this Path. We have to pay attention to how things are and have thoughts that reflect this understanding and do not, instead, distort reality. We have to be careful that our speech reflects clear thinking and understanding and creates harmony with others. We have to pay attention to our actions and make sure we conduct ourselves ethically and do not act is a way that unnecessarily increases our suffering or the suffering of others. That's a lot to keep in mind.

In the next chapters, we will explore the part of the Eightfold Path that cultivates mental discipline. It's hard to stay on course if we don't have mental discipline. We first will explore what is meant by Right Effort, or how we deal with using energy in our practice.

# Part IV

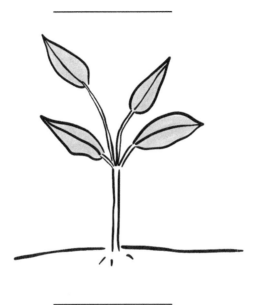

# Cultivating
# Mental Discipline

# 8

# RIGHT EFFORT

*"A disciplined mind leads to happiness,*
*and an undisciplined mind leads to suffering."*

*- Dalai Lama*

# Buddhism and Right Effort

Right Effort explores how we use energy in our practice. We derive it from the observation that, for something to happen, some effort must be expended to make it happen. Chance circumstance or the fairies will not magically deliver peace of mind to you. You must do it yourself. No one can do the work for you. Once we accept that we must make some kind of effort, how do we know what makes an effort "right?" We can gain a first hint if we recall the Buddhist notion of the Middle Way, of avoiding the suffering that derives from extremes.

Right Effort refers to attempting to cultivate wholesome qualities and eliminate unwholesome ones. It involves four aspects: preventing unwholesome states from arising, abandoning unwholesome states that have already arisen, cultivating wholesome states that have not yet arisen, and maintaining and enhancing wholesome states that have already arisen.

The Buddha used the analogy of a stringed musical instrument to explain Right Effort. If the string is too lax, it will not produce music. If too tight, it will break. The "music" comes from somewhere in between. If we don't try to make changes, practice, and pay attention, we may not achieve a positive result.

If we drive ourselves crazy trying to do everything at once, we contribute to suffering by trying too hard and not being in sync with how things are and how they are progressing. You can't go to the gym for the first time and, through the force of your will, decide that today you are going to bench press three hundred pounds. It would be best (and maybe essential!) to gradually work up to such a feat. Likewise, if you never go to the gym and challenge yourself, you will not develop.

Right Effort involves putting forth the necessary energy while being mindful of how things are. Along with being mindful, Right Effort also involves putting energy toward investigating how things are. If there is suffering or negative emotions, what are the conditions associated with this state? Sometimes I have to put in the effort to "connect the dots."

No one can always be perfectly mindful, but it is essential to return to this effort whenever negative states arise. Maybe I am putting forth much effort, but doing the wrong thing.

## The Five Hindrances

The Buddha said we must practice mental control. We achieve this mental control over time with systematic practice. Mental control prevents negative mental states from arising before they take hold. Within Buddhist philosophy, the five common ways this is thought to happen are called the five hindrances, or the five things that will undermine your efforts. The five hindrances are sensual desire, ill will, dullness, restlessness, and doubt.

*Sensual desire* means lust for pleasurable states of the body, food, sex, or for wealth, possessions, experiences, and accompanying pleasures. We all are capable of feeling pleasure. That is not a problem. The problem is when our mind wants to repeat that pleasure and strive for more; when this occurs, we become distracted and vulnerable to negative mental states. It is hard to see things clearly when focusing on desires. It is like adding dye that discolors a pool of water. The Buddha said a mind at ease will be like clear water reflecting your face.

*Ill will* means hatred, anger, resentment, and aversion, which are all states of mind that desire to reject something. If we practice hating, nurturing anger and resentment, and being judgmental or repulsing things, we become increasingly consumed by these states and attached to the ideas driving them. We then are so overcome with ill will that our efforts to move toward well-being are undermined. A mind in this state is sometimes described as frothy and boiling water. There is no clear reflection.

*Dullness* means mental inertia or fatigue, drowsiness, or general mental fogginess. A sleepy and dull mind cannot see things as they are. If water is overgrown with moss and algae, it cannot provide a clear reflection.

*Restlessness* refers to states of agitation or stress, which makes it difficult for the mind to focus. It is the state we too often experience in our modern life, in which many things capture our attention in a way that generates stress. If my mind is stressed and preoccupied, it is not in a state conducive to learning or growing emotionally. The Buddha described a restless mind as a pool of water stirred by the wind into ripples and waves.

*Doubt* means a mind full of questions and uncertainty, indecisive and lacking resolution. What if this happens? What if that happens? Is this the right thing? What is he thinking? If my mind is busy with questions and fear, it is hard to see things as they are. This is like murky water – like a cloudy suspension that has been placed in a dark place – you can't see through it here either.

# CBT and Right Effort

CBT is also an endeavor that requires some effort. Most CBT activities involve practicing the concepts and tools. It is essential to do your homework!

Exposure-based treatments for anxiety entail actively moving toward things that cue anxiety. Learning how to change thought patterns reflective of cognitive distortions requires regular journal writing to get in the habit of being mindful of thought patterns. If we approach the process passively, it is not likely that much change will happen. Effective learning is an active process rather than a passive one.

At the end of a therapy visit, it has long been my habit to say something like: "See you next week. Enjoy the rest of your day, and *have good practice.*" Like most anything in life, we get good at what we practice. If I practice being angry, I will get good at it. If I practice worrying, I will get good at it. Communicate using the Four Horsemen (see chapter 5, Right Speech) every day and you will eventually become a master.

If I practice ignoring the consequences of my actions, I will become good at it. It is hard sometimes to see our difficulties as the result of ways of thinking or acting that we have practiced. We tend to think that our difficulties occur because of chance circumstances. *"Out there" is making me feel . . . I certainly have no choice in how I react. That's just who I am.* It is vital to understand this tendency and apply effort more skillfully.

## Process-oriented Frame vs. Goal-oriented Frame

There are many definitions for what it means to be process-oriented. It generally refers to having a system and focusing on following the system rather than the goal itself. A *process orientation* still relates to a goal. The process is how I arrive at the goal. The goal is the destination.

We are often taught to set goals and work hard to achieve them. The problem with this *goal-oriented frame* is that it doesn't necessarily give you a better result, and it can make the process of getting there less exciting or fun because your focus is on the destination. *I will be happy just as soon as I arrive at the goal.*

Thomas Sterner, founder and CEO of The Practicing Mind Institute, explains how being overly goal-oriented when learning a new skill causes anxiety surrounding the activity. If I focus on the goal instead of the practice, I cannot be in the present moment, because my attention is on the distance between my current ability and the ability I wish to achieve. Measuring in this way makes practice an unpleasant experience, leading people to avoid doing it because of how it makes them feel (Sterner, 2012). This dynamic is unfortunate, as practice is the only way to improve at anything. Even if I can apply discipline and overcome this feeling, I don't experience the joy of working toward the goal. Then I discover that when I arrive at the finish line, I am no happier, or if I am, it is only briefly. I then reset toward another goal and keep chasing that same elusive happiness. *I will be happy just as soon as . . .*

Learning anything involves practice. Practice can be defined as "the deliberate repetition of a process with the intention of reaching a specific goal" (Sterner, 2012). But we tend to see the process of practice as a "necessary nuisance we have to go through to get to our goal." When we view the process this way, we will probably become bored, frustrated, and impatient, or even discouraged.

To enjoy the process, we need to become more present-minded, focusing on the immediate experience without the pressure of the ultimate goal. For example, I can reach my ultimate goal of becoming skilled at jiujitsu by simply practicing that objective during this training session and the next. As the months and years go by, I realize I am becoming more skilled and progressing in the art. When we approach the process in this way, there isn't any pressure because our primary goal is "to pay attention to only what I am doing now," so that you are "achieving your goal in each and every moment," as Sterner puts it.

"This process brings us inner peace and a wonderful sense of mastery and self-confidence. We are mastering ourselves by staying in the process and mastering whatever activity we work on. This is the essence of proper practice" (Sterner, 2012).

Having goals and a process that carries you effectively toward them is good. It is also helpful to have activities that you pursue not so much for the purpose of arriving at a destination, but because the process is an end unto itself. Art forms and hobbies are examples of this idea. You never really master a martial art. There are always areas to improve and new things to learn. But with practice, the art form is understood more fully. Likewise, if I play guitar or another musical instrument, I never truly master it. There is always more to learn. Suppose I love to paint. I will never paint all the pictures or master all the techniques. Art forms and hobbies help us to understand it is not always about reaching a goal.

If I have a goal that is detached from a process, I am more at risk of drifting from the goal. Let's say I have a goal to "get healthier," but I don't establish a process to take me toward that goal. I might have a salad for lunch today instead of a cheeseburger. I might go for a run or lift some weights. I might faithfully do similar things each day for the next few weeks. Then one day, I have a flat tire and need to spend the afternoon dealing with it, so I don't go for a run that day. The next day, I have lunch with a friend at that excellent burger place. Being stuffed from lunch, I don't feel like running that afternoon. The following weekend, relatives are visiting. Gradually, one thing or another distracts me. I have good intentions and I follow through whenever I think of the goal. But slowly, more and more of everyday life competes for my attention. Pretty soon, I am no longer focused on my goal of being healthy.

Contrast this with a process-oriented frame. I decide to "get healthier." I think about a process (a recurrent activity over time) that is logically connected to the goal. For each meal, I might minimize carbs and increase my intake of vegetables. Every Monday, Wednesday, Friday, and Sunday, I will go on a thirty-minute run. I set up the process and let the outcome take care of itself. But if I don't have a process, I will likely lose my connection with the goal that was once important to me.

## Motivation vs. Discipline

Motivation is having the desire to do something. We might be motivated to do something that is enjoyable or rewarding, or because it meets a vital need. I need to be healthy, so I am motivated to exercise. I want more opportunities in life, so I pursue an education. I want to make a million dollars, so I work hard in my business. Motivations are as varied as people are varied.

The problem with motivation is that it often waxes and wanes. Some days we just "don't feel like it." In this case, what to do?

Well, first, it is good to listen to your body. Is it giving you the message you need to rest and recover? Are you approaching burnout or excessive mental fatigue? If so, heed that message. But if there is no good reason not to do the planned activity, then you may need to practice discipline.

Discipline is when you continue doing what is necessary, whether or not you are motivated. It keeps us on course toward what is important to us. Discipline is when I go to training anyway, even if I'm not motivated. What I have found interesting is that when I use discipline to stay on course regardless of my level of motivation, I usually feel better. Rarely have I regretted going to training.

It is a misconception that disciplined individuals are those who are constantly grinding and never have any fun. Research has shown that people with high self-control are happier than those with less self-control, because the self-disciplined people are more capable of dealing with goal conflicts. They spend less time debating whether to indulge in behaviors detrimental to their health and can make beneficial decisions more easily. The self-disciplined do not allow their choices to be dictated by impulses or feelings. Instead, they make informed, rational decisions daily without feeling overly stressed or upset. When I take this approach, I wind up being happier because I achieve more of the things that are important to me.

Your motivation will inevitably wax and wane. Understanding this helps you to use discipline to stay on course. Remember, you are working toward something that you have said is important. If you remain consistent, even though your motivation waxes and wanes, you will eventually arrive at the desired result. This makes you happy! If you veer off course or give up altogether and never achieve the result—how happy will you be?

Improving self-discipline means changing routine behaviors, which can be uncomfortable initially. Charles Duhigg, the author of *The Power of Habit*, explains that habitual behaviors are traced to a part of the brain called the basal ganglia, which is associated with emotions, patterns, and memories. Conscious decisions, on the other hand, are made in the prefrontal cortex, a completely different area. When a behavior becomes a habit, we stop using our decision-making skills and instead function on autopilot (Duhigg, 2014). Therefore, if I follow a process, such as training every Wednesday, Friday, and Saturday, over time the process becomes a habit. *Oh, it's Friday, time to train.* Why are you training? *Because it's Friday.*

Breaking a bad habit and building a new one requires us to make active decisions, and it will also feel wrong. Your brain will resist the change in favor of what it has already been programmed to do. When developing a new habit, it is helpful to use a technique called "habit stacking" (Duhigg, 2014). Even the most undisciplined of us still have some things that we do regularly, such as working out, taking the dog for a walk, brushing our teeth, eating dinner, and the like.

If you want to develop a new habit, you increase your chance of success by pairing it with an existing habit. For example, if you wanted to become more disciplined about meditating, you might pair it with eating breakfast. *I am allowed to eat breakfast after I have meditated for ten minutes.* When you do this, the new habit "inherits" some of the habit force of the existing habit.

You may be motivated to achieve various goals, but discipline is what will keep you focused on the process carrying you toward them. Remember what Yoda said: "Do. Or do not. There is no try."

## Exploring Limits

Part of discerning Right Effort is exploring one's limits. What are my limits? How much effort should I put toward this task? Is this my actual limit, or is it a self-imposed one rooted in doubt? The Navy Seals have the "40% Rule." This rule refers to the idea that we have a safety breaker hardwired into us. When we are physically and mentally spent and think, *I am at my limit. I cannot go on,* this thought is just a buffer that mother nature put in our brain so we don't hurt ourselves. Realistically, however, when we first start having these thoughts, we have only used about forty percent of our actual capacity. Our minds say, "Stop. This is all I can do." However, if you override this reflex, you will discover much more capacity beyond that point. This idea might also apply to when we feel psychologically spent.

I experienced a sense of pushing my limits from running. I started out as a jogger, usually running two to four miles a few times a week to stay in good condition. Then I explored my limits, wondering how far I might run. Gradually I decided to try a marathon, which is twenty-six miles. Realizing I could accomplish that, I wanted to see if I could take it farther. So I started running ultramarathons, which are fifty to a hundred miles long. These endurance exercises are as much mental as physical. It feels as though you are at your limit, but then you test that limit to see if it is real or imagined. The actual limit differs from the perceived limit, and both can change from day to day.

A few years ago, my youngest daughter asked me if I'd like to do a Tough Mudder race with her. I said, "Sure. What's a Tough Mudder?" She explained that it's race whose proceeds go to the Wounded

Warrior Foundation. It is about twelve miles long and, as the name implies, it's about ninety percent mud. To make it more fun, obstacles are placed every quarter mile along the course. Many are ones you might picture on boot camp training courses. Others are things like ice water immersion or mud pits with electrical wires to avoid or get a rather noticeable shock. There are wooden walls six to twelve feet high, many of which it's not possible to scale alone. You have to rely on another racer to stop at the top and give you a hand, and sometimes you also need a shove up from below.

I quickly realized that no matter your age, how tough you are, or how athletic you are, you cannot finish a Tough Mudder race by yourself. You require help from other racers, or you will stand alone in front of a wall you cannot scale. Like most people, I often live in the illusion of being self-contained and self-reliant. However, in a Buddhist framework, we are reminded of the reality that we are interdependent. I often think about that day and am reminded how our individual accomplishments are often the result of our interdependence with others. Sometimes we can push our limits a little further with the support of others.

When I was promoted to black belt in jiujitsu, I recalled the Tough Mudder race and the feeling of interdependence. I had the same feeling about receiving the black belt. In some respects, it is certainly an individual achievement. You must train consistently, struggle with the challenges and discomforts, and push yourself to where your instructor sees your progress as worthy of a black belt. You must do the work; the fairies won't do it for you. You must exert Right Effort. However, nobody gets there alone. You must have training partners. They must work with you, provide feedback, encouragement, and challenges, and "give you a hand up to overcome obstacles." Teachers must share their knowledge and guide your development. Because of this interdependence, it is a group effort when someone achieves the rank of black belt.

Is exploring limits in the service of the ego? It can be if one is not careful. The important thing is to ask yourself is whether you are exploring limits as part of your self-growth and understanding, or to be admired by others and enhance your ego. If you do things in the service of the ego, you fall into the perpetual problem of measuring. Yes, I ran a marathon. I feel good when I think of that and feel satisfaction when people admire that achievement. However, my marathon times were far below average compared to other marathoners. I have run ultramarathons. Not many people can do that. However, I also run ultramarathons very slowly compared to "real" ultramarathon athletes.

I am a black belt in jiujitsu. I have been a world champion several times over in my age division. However, other black belts at my school are also world champions in younger, more competitive divisions and could easily overcome me as if I were a beginner. We always run into the measuring problem when it is about ego. Who or what am I comparing my ego to? *Compared to this—I come out great. Compared to that—meh, not so much.* In practicing Right Effort we ask ourselves, *How was that experience? What did I learn?* Measuring the experience instead of the self is a very different mindset.

An ego-driven motivation is primarily focused on enhancing one's self-image or sense of importance in the eyes of others. This type of motivation is often based on external validation and recognition and may involve comparing oneself to others, seeking approval or admiration, or avoiding failure or criticism.

In contrast, growth-driven motivation primarily focuses on personal development, learning, and self-improvement. This type of motivation is often based on internal standards and values and may involve taking on challenges, seeking new experiences, or learning from mistakes or failures. It's important to note that these motivations are not mutually exclusive, and it's possible to have a mix of ego-driven and growth-driven motivations at different times or in different situations. However, cultivating a growth-driven motivation can lead to greater personal fulfillment, resilience, and long-term success, as it is based on internal values and personal growth rather than external validation or comparison to others.

There is nothing wrong with striving for a goal and then being content once we achieve it. However, occasionally, it is good to go a bit further and explore your limits—not to serve the ego or chase satisfaction outside of yourself, but rather to step outside of the ego and test your limits through actual experience of them. There are often many facets of our ego where we limit ourselves. We tell ourselves things like, *Oh, I could never do that.* That might be so, but have you tested that belief against your direct experience?

We can explore our limits in any realm, not solely the physical. Whatever you do, can you do a little more or go a little farther? This effort can break down notions you hold about who you are. Examine some things you already do and then ask yourself if you could go a little farther. Can you try something you have never done before and see how the experience unfolds?

## Consistency vs. Intensity

If you want to achieve a goal that is very difficult and requires a lot of effort, there are two ways you might go about it. One is consistency and the other is intensity.

Let's use an example of a ultramarathon race (50+ miles) approached with intensity. I decide to sign up for the race. I am super motivated and psyched to complete it. As training, I decide I am going to run twenty miles every day as fast as I can. With this approach, probably in less than a week I will have a major injury or my motivation will exhaust itself.

The second option is consistency. I have the same goal; however, I go about reaching it in a different way. I do some research and discover that people who have completed such races follow a pattern of consistent training that usually starts with low mileage that increases gradually and is punctuated with regular rest and recovery days. Following this pattern, I train consistently, and then race day takes care of itself.

Intensity soon burns out. Consistency leads to steady progress toward the desired outcome.

There is an old story about a new student at a karate school who asked his instructor how long it would take to get a black belt. The instructor answered that it might take four to five years. The student said, "What if I train five days a week?" The instructor said, "Maybe six or seven years." The student said, "What if I train every day, including weekends? How long will it take?" The instructor said, "Probably ten to twelve years." The student, now puzzled, asked, "What if I dedicate myself to training and train several times a day, every day? How long will it take?" The instructor replied, "You will probably never achieve a black belt." The student, now very frustrated, asked why. The instructor replied, "With all of your focus on the destination, you will not have any focus left for the journey."

How do you achieve a long endeavor like a college education? It's the same principle. You consistently attend class, complete your homework each day, study for the test, finish the course, and repeat. With consistent application of effort, you eventually arrive at the destination. The focus of your effort is on the day-to-day. Part of the irony of consistency over intensity is that if I approach an endeavor with consistency, I am in a better position to make an intense effort for a short time. Consistency enables intensity.

## Effort and Outcome

Right Effort involves making a sustained effort to cultivate wholesome states of mind and abandon unwholesome states of mind. In this context, it may seem counterintuitive to think that one could have Right Effort and still experience a bad outcome. However, it is important to remember that the outcome of any effort is not entirely within our control but is influenced by a complex array of factors.

Our understanding of what makes up a "bad" outcome may not always be accurate, as sometimes unexpected difficulties can lead to valuable learning experiences and growth. In this way, the focus of Right Effort is not necessarily on the outcome, but on the intention and effort put into the action. By exerting Right Effort, a person can cultivate positive habits and mindsets that can help them navigate difficult situations and overcome obstacles, even if the outcome is not what they hoped for. So while a "bad" outcome may occur, the practice of Right Effort can still lead to personal growth, resilience, compassion, wisdom, and a greater sense of well-being.

We want to be mindful of how we are expendin our efforts. Right Effort should support our journey toward cultivating a peaceful mind and a feeling of contentment. It is important to realize that.

Something important to remember with Right Effort is that sometimes we can put in a great deal of effort but toward the wrong thing. For example, I might be a kind, giving person and put much effort into practicing that. However, I might put all this effort into a narcissist who will never be satisfied, no matter how giving I am. I might train hard, be in good condition, do everything anyone could ask someone to do to prepare for a competition, then get caught in a choke.

The coach of the football team might call for exactly the correct play, the team might execute it perfectly, but the touchdown does not happen. I might work hard, do everything to complete my work effectively but still not get the promotion because the boss's nephew did. There are always other factors at play besides our own individual effort.

## The Path Forward . . .

To walk the Path effectively takes mental discipline. Part of mental discipline is the effort we put forth. Right Effort follows the Middle Way. We can't be passive in our practice and expect results. It also does no good to drive ourselves crazy trying too hard. We want to stay focused, not getting distracted by desires or angry thoughts. We don't want to allow ourselves to be lazy, filled with restlessness, or caught up in questions that have no answers. We want to understand that our motivation will wax and wane and that's okay, because discipline will keep us on course. Steady, consistent progress will get us there more reliably than intense bursts of effort. Making sure our efforts are effectively focused requires a combination of concentration and mindfulness which we will explore next.

# 9

# RIGHT CONCENTRATION

*Keep it simple and focus on what matters.*
*Don't let yourself be overwhelmed.*

*- Confuscius*

# Buddhism and Right Concentration

The practice of Right Concentration is to cultivate a mind that is one-pointed. In Buddhism there are commonly understood to be two kinds of concentration: *active* and *selective*. Sometimes our mind will dwell on whatever is happening in the present moment as it changes. This is called active concentration.

Selective concentration entails choosing one object and holding onto it. We are aware of whatever else is happening, but our focus is on the object. Mindfulness is being aware of our direct experience in the present moment without judging that moment harshly. I may be mindful that a lot is happening around me or that my mind is busy with dozens of thoughts. When I am mindful of everything going on, I use selective concentration to focus on one thing. This one object of focus becomes the foreground, and all the rest becomes background.

Selective concentration or one-pointed focus is part of Right Concentration, but more is needed. It must be connected to Right Understanding to cultivate a useful state of mind. For example, if I have a single-minded focus but use it to avoid my problems or escape the reality of my situation, I am practicing an unhealthy state of mind. In this case, I am practicing dissociation. I am concentrating on some-thing in order to "zone out" so I won't have the face the thing that troubles me. This is not a sound practice if my one-pointed focus is on an unwholesome state of mind, such as ill will or revenge. If I have a one-pointed focus but lose my sense of mindfulness about what is going on, I may be doing less than optimal practice. A soldier on the battlefield may have a one-pointed focus as well. So will an assassin about to slay a victim. These examples reflect a concentrated mind but not Right Concentration.

The Buddha compared a mind without concentration to a flapping fish taken out of the water and thrown onto dry land. Such a mind flies from one thought to another without inner control. This lack of concentration makes one vulnerable to worries and concerns generated by random thoughts. A mind that has practiced Right Concentration can remain focused without distraction. This ability to focus allows one to achieve a state where the mind is a more accurate mirror of how things are.

If Right Concentration is a focus on a wholesome object that creates clarity, what might wrong concentration be? The practice of the Eightfold Path trains the mind to focus on healthy, tranquil, and compassionate states, in order to cultivate a mind that practices the cessation of suffering for ourselves and others. Wrong concentration would be concentration that does not have this aim. An assassin may be skilled and able to concentrate on their objective, but the concentration is not compassionate. As we cultivate Right Concentration, we should ensure it aligns with Right Understanding and Right Thought. Is our calm, concentrated mind also intent on developing loving-kindness and compassion for others?

A one-pointed focus is developed by a regular *meditation practice*. Meditation is a mental exercise for developing certain mental skills. It is not about achieving some weird, altered mental state, but about practicing the cultivation of an ordinary mental process that supports our well-being and our journey on the Eightfold Path. It can strengthen the ability to focus and concentrate and promote greater mindfulness (see chapter 10) and self-awareness. By practicing meditation regularly, we can develop greater control over our thoughts and emotions and become more aware of how our thought patterns and behaviors influence our mental state and overall well-being.

# CBT and Right Concentration

In CBT, Right Concentration can be understood as the ability to direct one's attention and thoughts toward a specific goal or task and maintain that focus despite distractions or obstacles.

In addition to meditation practice, we could develop habits and practices that promote greater concentration and focus, such as setting clear goals and priorities, establishing routines and schedules, and engaging in regular exercise and other physical activity.

Ultimately, the goal of developing Right Concentration is to improve our ability to focus and direct mental energy to promote greater clarity, mindfulness, and self-awareness. In Buddhism, "wrong concentration" is often understood as mental fixation or obsession characterized by a lack of mindfulness, clarity, and insight. In CBT, this might be understood as mental inflexibility or rigidity characterized by a lack of adaptability and problem-solving ability.

For example, if you are practicing meditation or trying to develop Right Concentration, a few signs may show that you are experiencing "wrong concentration." You may become fixated on a particular thought or sensation to the point that it becomes difficult to shift your focus. You may feel agitated or restless rather than calm and focused.

Becoming overly critical or judgmental of yourself or others rather than cultivating a sense of compassion and equanimity may also be a sign. You may feel disconnected from your body or surroundings rather than being fully present in the moment.

Remember that the practice of meditation and Right Concentration is a journey, and it is normal to experience challenges and setbacks along the way. By remaining open, flexible, and compassionate, you can continue to grow and develop your practice.

## The Myth of Multitasking

Multitasking refers to trying to perform multiple tasks simultaneously or in rapid succession. We might be driving, listening to a podcast, or scanning Facebook while talking on the phone. We might be engaged with a work project while also checking email. At home, we might be making dinner, listening to the news, and helping the kids with homework. The idea is that by doing multiple tasks simultaneously, one can increase efficiency and productivity.

However, recent research has shown that the human brain cannot multitask. This rapid switching can lead to decreased productivity and increased errors, as the brain cannot focus fully on any one task. One study found that when people attempt to multitask, their performance on all tasks is worse than if they had focused on one task at a time. Multitasking can also negatively affect our emotional state, increasing stress and anxiety and leading to a sense of overwhelm. One study found that multitasking can activate the body's stress response, negatively affecting physical and mental health (Mehta et al., 2016). It's better to focus on one task at a time and complete it before moving on to the next one.

We have a tendency to inflate our perceived ability to multitask. Studies have shown little correlation between our belief in being able to multitask and our actual ability. Multitasking is almost always a misnomer. Our brains are constructed with a bias toward single-task focus. The brain structures related to attention and executive control make it difficult if not impossible for us to truly multitask. When we attempt to multitask, usually what we are actually doing is rapidly switching between one task and another (Madore & Wagner, 2019).

If I believe I am a champion multitasker, I probably am not practicing Right Concentration. I will be fooling myself into believing that I am doing three or four things at once. I will also overestimate how great I am at doing this juggling. If I do two things at once, the brain will divide the attentional resources devoted to each task in half.

## Right Concentration in the Age of Information Overload

The internet contains more information than all the world's libraries combined. An almost incomprehensibly vast volume of information is available to us via a few keystrokes in the query box of a search engine. However, much of this information can be wrong or misleading. It behooves us to consume information only after exercising due diligence with critical thinking. However, our ability to exert attention and concentration to sort through the search results can be overcome by overwhelm.

To make information management more workable, Kozyreva and colleagues (2022) advocate *critical ignoring*, which is "the ability to choose what to ignore and where to invest one's limited attentional capacities. Critical ignoring is more than just not paying attention—it's about practicing mindful and healthy habits in the face of information overabundance. It is a core competence for all citizens in the digital world. Without it, we will drown in a sea of information that is, at best, distracting and, at worst, misleading and harmful." They describe three key strategies for practicing critical ignoring. Each corresponds to a particular type of noxious information.

1. *Self-nudging:* This strategy aims to control the type and manner of exposure to the information environment. It might entail turning off notifications or setting specific time aside to check emails, to create pockets of distraction-free concentration. Self-nudging helps us avoid constant information updating— checking texts, email, Facebook, Instagram, news feeds, and so on repeatedly during the day.

2. *Lateral reading*: The second strategy involves opening a new browser tab to search for information about the organization or individual behind a site to check the credibility of the source before diving into its contents. Many sites can be deceptive unless you are an expert in that field. They can have a slick interface and appear to be quoting "studies" or "experts" when they are actually peddling misinformation. Most sites thrive on attention, views, and clicks to generate revenue. Save attentional resources by first vetting the source.

3. *Resist engaging with trolls*: The last strategy is to apply the do-not-feed-the-trolls heuristic. Trolls thrive on attention, and deliberate spreaders of dangerous disinformation often resort to trolling tactics. One of science denialists' main strategies is to hijack people's attention by creating the appearance of debate when none exists. The heuristic advises not to respond to trolls. Resist debating or retaliating. Reserve your attentional resources for other, more productive uses.

## Mind vs. Brain

Training the mind to have sustained focused concentration is a good practice on the Path. We have minds, but our minds live in a brain. Not all brains are the same.

It is important to note that some disorders have distinct neuro-chemical components that can compromise the ability to have focused attention and concentrate. For example, attention deficit hyperactivity disorder (ADHD) is a syndrome that is characterized by age-inappro-priate inattention, hyperactivity, and impulsivity.

Medication is the primary treatment for both children and adults with ADHD. Stimulants are the most common type of prescription medication used to treat ADHD. They don't work by increasing stim-ulation. Instead, they work by increasing levels of certain chemicals (neurotransmitters) in the brain called dopamine and norepinephrine. These neurotransmitters play an essential role in paying attention and staying motivated. Many studies have shown that, on average, about eighty percent of children with ADHD have fewer symptoms once prescribed the correct medication and dosage.

Another disorder that can have a neurochemical component that affects concentration is depression. Depression is a mental disorder that varies from mild to severe. When severe, various brain functions can be disrupted, including those that regulate sleep, appetite, mood, and concentration. A PET scan can identify distinct differences in brain activity during periods of depression when compared to normal brain activity.

Like ADHD, severe depression is sometimes treated with medication and other interventions. These treatments try to stimulate neurotrans-mitters in the brain, such as serotonin, dopamine, and norepinephrine. Both CBT and antidepressant treatments can cause observable changes in brain functioning, although in different areas. Antidepressants have been shown to evoke neural changes in the neighborhood of the amygdala, whereas psychotherapy evokes anatomically distinct differences in the medial prefrontal cortex. Both psychotherapy- and antidepressant-related changes converged on regions of the emotional regulation network. These findings may account for the research that shows both CBT and antidepressant treatments to be effective, but a combined treatment to have additional benefits.

This brain-mind connection related to concentration is also observed in other serious mental illnesses, such as bipolar disorder and schizophrenia. Brain diseases such as various dementias can impact the ability to concentrate. Medical conditions like low vitamin D or B12 or hypothyroidism can also negatively affect concentration. Recent research is currently exploring "brain fog" associated with long COVID.

The point of this discussion is to remember that you have a mind, but your mind lives in a brain. The influences can move in both directions. You can change your behaviors and mental practices, creating observable physical changes in your brain. The brain can also become imbalanced, impacting mental processes such as concentration and other functions usually thought to be strictly in the realm of the "mind." If you have one of the disorders discussed here, consult an appropriate professional. If properly treated, the resulting mental functions can improve, your concentration can improve, and you can continue your journey along the Path.

## Task Management System

It is common that when someone has trouble concentrating, they often have a pattern of holding things in their mind and then continually processing them out of fear of forgetting them. Unless we are blessed with a photographic memory, our mind has limited bandwidth to hold things in memory.

When we consider our entire to-do list at once, we can feel overwhelmed. However, we can only *do* one thing at a time. Practicing Right Concentration means staying connected to this reality. I can be mindful that I have many things to do, but I concentrate instead with a focused mind on what I am doing now. If I am overwhelmed, it is usually because I am wandering around in my head, repeatedly replaying the list. I am disconnected from the task at hand. It is important to use the feeling of being overwhelmed to alert you that you have lost Right Concentration. Once you notice that, you can shift focus to the task you are doing.

A useful tool to support concentrated focus is a task management or to-do list system. The method you use can be simple or complex, old school or digital, but it needs to be functional. I remember visiting with a patient who ran a large, successful company he built from the ground up. He kept an index card in his front pocket. On one side were his scheduled activities, and on the other was his list of tasks for the day. Low-tech, and very functional. Another patient was a middle-level manager who had a fancy planner with all sorts of pages and a color-coded lists that he frequently updated. Despite this, he felt perpetually behind, overwhelmed, and anxious. His system was complicated, but not functional.

To start a task management system, first, do a "mind dump." Write down *everything* that you feel you need to do, either today or someday. Get used to getting stuff out of your head and into the system. Because you are just one person, I encourage you to have a single system that includes work and personal tasks. Having an integrated list helps to weigh priorities among the spheres of your life.

It is essential to link tasks with time. For each task, ask yourself *when* you will do the task. If you have just a long list of tasks with no scheduling, you are more likely to become overwhelmed, which does not create ideal conditions for concentrated focus. Each morning, take tasks from the master list and create a plan for the day. At the end of the day, review how the plan went and rearrange tasks accordingly. The process takes just a few minutes in the morning and again in the evening.

Sometimes you may have trouble concentrating, not because you keep replaying your to-do list in your head, but because you are replaying something that is troubling you. In this case, you may find relief by journaling—writing a narrative about what is troubling you often helps to ease rumination. It is almost as if the mind says, "There is a hard copy, so I guess I can stop recycling these thoughts." Extending the journaling with the 3-column technique discussed in chapter 4 is even better.

## Flow State

People I train with at my jiujitsu school know I am a psychologist. Because of that, I occasionally get asked about anxiety. Years ago, if someone had asked me if jiujitsu training would suit someone with anxiety, I probably would have said it might worsen it. Jiujitsu is a grappling martial art. Your training partner attempts to get hold of you, take you to the ground, attain a physically dominant position over you , and then compel you to submit via a choke or joint lock. You would think that if you are anxious about everyday life things, then the last activity you would pursue would be a sport that is a symbolic fight to the death. If your opponent gets you in a choke hold, you tap three times, and they release. You usually smile and say something like "Good one!" slap hands, fist bump, and go at it again.

I have found the positive effect of this martial art on anxiety very interesting. There are many accounts of people with general stress and anxiety and of soldiers or police officers with PTSD benefiting from this activity. I have had several instances of people taking me aside, telling me about their struggles with anxiety, and asking if it was weird that the *only* time they *don't* feel anxious is when they are training.

A five-month study on the effect of juijitsu training on veterans suffering from PTSD found clinically significant improvements in symptoms of PTSD, as well as meaningful reductions in PTSD-associated syndromes, including depression, generalized anxiety, and alcohol use. The magnitude of the effect sizes suggests that routine practice of Brazilian jiujitsu (BJJ) may be a beneficial complementary approach for treating PTSD (Willing et al., 2019).

A review of the academic literature on the effects of BBJ training on participants showed that it holds promise as a beneficial psychological intervention. It is consistently associated with low levels of aggression, the development of resilience, and the possibility of extending one's social network. BJJ may offer a community that can buffer against mental illness and promote well-being.

An activity like BJJ is conducive to what is sometimes called a "flow state." People can experience flow during all sorts of situations. These can include games like chess, sports like basketball or jiujitsu, professional activities like performing surgery, or creative activities like painting or playing a musical instrument.

In his book *Finding Flow*, Mihaly Csikszentmihalyi (1997) described several aspects necessary for a flow state:

- A clear set of goals that require clear responses
- Immediate feedback
- A balance between the task and one's skill level so that the challenge is not too high or too low
- Complete focus on the task
- A lack of self-consciousness

- The distortion of time, such that time seems to pass more quickly than usual
- The feeling that the activity is intrinsically rewarding
- A sense of strength and control over the task

There are interesting changes that happen in the brain during a flow state. Activity in the prefrontal cortex is decreased. This area of the brain handles complex cognitive functions, including include memory, monitoring time, and self-consciousness. In a process called *hypofrontality*, the prefrontal cortex is temporarily inhibited, which likely causes the time distortion and lack of self-consciousness a person experiences when in a flow state. Decreased activity in the prefrontal cortex enables more accessible communication between other areas of the brain, and as a result, the mind is more creative. A flow state has many benefits, such as improved performance and increased happiness.

Different activities facilitate a flow state for different people. While one person may enter a flow state while tending to flowers, another may do so while drawing or running an ultramarathon. The key is to find an activity you are passionate about and enjoy. It should also have a specific goal and a method to achieve that goal.

The activity must be challenging enough to require you to push the limits of your skill level just a little beyond your current capabilities. The balance between skill level and challenge must be optimal to cause deep involvement in the activity and create the desired flow state. If the challenge too greatly exceeds current skill levels, it can lead to frustration and anxiety. However if it is too easy, it can lead to boredom. A flow state requires a concentrated focus. Smartphones and other distractions must be removed to achieve a flow state.

*Mushin no shin* is a Japanese martial art concept that translates to "mind of no mind." It refers to a state of mind where the practitioner is fully present in the moment and can react without conscious thought or distraction. This state is achieved through discipline, training, and a deep understanding of one's thoughts and emotions, and it allows for fluid, intuitive movements in response to any situation. Cultivating *mushin no shin* is one way of practicing Right Concentration.

The concepts of flow state and *mushin no shin* share similarities in that they both describe a mental state in which the individual is fully immersed in the present moment and can perform at their best without distraction or conscious thought.

Regular physical training in specific techniques helps to build muscle memory and develop the ability to respond instinctively to different situations. Mindfulness and meditation can help you become aware of thoughts and emotions and develop greater control over them. Letting go of the desire for personal gain or recognition (ego) can help to stay focused and respond without hesitation or distraction. In training, repetition helps with confronting and overcoming fears, which in turn builds confidence and the ability to remain calm and focused under pressure. Spending an hour of training with someone trying to choke you unconscious just seems to make the rest of the day seem manageable.

## The Path Forward . . .

Our practice along the Path is enhanced when we can focus on one thing while still being aware of all the other things going on. Concentration and mindfulness complement one another. It is important to have a focused mind, but the focus should support a wholesome state of mind. Our brains can sometimes have trouble with concentration, but can be influenced by our mental practices. We can have behavioral habits that can support concentration or lead us to be perpetually distracted.

While concentration is an intentional awareness of a single object, mindfulness is a more diffuse awareness of all that is going on at any given moment. In the next chapter we will explore mindfulness and how to cultivate this mental skill.

# 10

# RIGHT MINDFULNESS

*If you are depressed, you are living in the past.*
*If you are anxious, you are living in the future.*
*If you are at peace, you are living in the present.*

*Lao Tsu*

# Buddhism and Right Mindfulness

Mindfulness is the basis for all the other components on the Path. We notice how each component of the Eightfold Path complements the others. Unless one is mindful, it is hard to maintain an awareness of Right View, Thought, Speech, Action, Livelihood, Effort, or Concentration.

Mindfulness is a type of attention. It is a mental state of being present and fully engaged in the current moment, with an open and non-judgmental awareness of one's thoughts, feelings, and surroundings. It involves paying deliberate attention to one's experiences, including sensations in the body, emotions, and thoughts, without becoming lost in them or reacting to them impulsively.

Most everyone has had experiences that are mindful. An example might be a time when you stepped outside and saw an awesome sunset that took your breath away. For just a moment, you were completely absorbed in the experience of gazing at the beautiful colors. Or you might have been completely absorbed in the experience of listening to your favorite song. Or you were sitting in a park and not really thinking about anything in particular, just feeling the breeze on your face, soaking up the sunshine and watching the squirrels play.

For most of us, the experience is accidental, yet it's so engaging that we immediately connect to it and get out of our noisy heads, if only for a moment. We may notice that when we are in a mindful state, we are unselfconscious, feel relaxed, and our minds feel quiet and centered. It would be great to spend all day in the park with the squirrels and top it off with a magnificent sunset. Watch sunsets every day—but who has the time? Right?

What we don't often realize is that mindfulness is a mental state that can be cultivated intentionally in a variety of ways. Gradually, with practice, we can learn to be mindful on demand. We can learn how to be in that state without the help of an awesome sunset or cute scampering squirrels. We can learn to shift into that mode whenever it is useful to do so. Practically, we might reflect on whether we are mindful of loved ones or even ourselves. For example, we might ask, *Am I fully listening to my partner or my child when they are speaking or am I distracted by things in my surroundings or in my mind? Am I fully present while I am eating my meal, or do I look down and wonder who ate my lunch?*

Developing this skill is very much worth the effort. In a Buddhist framework, mindfulness has long been noted as an important element of the Eightfold Path. In modern psychology, is has been found to be a very important component to mental health. Mindfulness is often cultivated through various forms of mindfulness-based meditation, but it can also be incorporated into daily activities, such as walking, eating, or interacting with others. By practicing mindfulness, we can develop greater clarity, focus, and emotional resilience, and reduce stress and anxiety. We can then use mindfulness off and on during the day whenever it is useful.

## Basic Meditation Practice

Meditation is an ancient practice that has been studied scientifically in recent decades. With advancements in brain scanning technology, we can now see what happens in the brain as a result of this basic mental practice. We now know that meditation can rewire connections in the brain. There is downregulation in parts of the brain associated with stress and threats and upregulation in the area of the brain associated with feelings of well-being. And the more one practices, the stronger these changes.

Meditation practice does not aim to change your thoughts. The practice is to change how you relate to your thoughts. Your mind is always thinking thoughts like your lungs are always breathing breaths. This mental activity is a constant mix of plans, memories, feelings, impressions, intentions, deep thoughts, and trivial thoughts. It is constant, much like a stream of water, and is in fact sometimes referred to as *the thought stream.*

However, one part of this stream differs from all the rest. That is awareness. Our minds can think of stuff and, at the same time, be aware that we are thinking stuff. Awareness is separate and apart from all the rest. The mind has one part that thinks stuff and another that observes what it is thinking.

Awareness has two important qualities: *voluntary* and *involuntary.* To some extent, it is under our voluntary control. Much like a flashlight, we can point awareness wherever we like. The light beam can be narrow like a laser or diffuse like a lamp. A second quality of awareness is that it can also be involuntarily captured and redirected. If there is a sudden noise outside, you will instantly forget what you are doing and focus on the unexpected event. If something triggers a memory with a strong emotion attached to it, your awareness might be captured for a moment by this internal event. Having more voluntary control over awareness is associated with well-being. Less control over awareness is associated with more stress and emotional reactivity.

So, how do we develop more control over awareness? That is where meditation practice comes in. It is like exercising a muscle. You do repetitions of an exercise, and the muscle strengthens. Here, we want to strengthen a mental muscle. As you have done earlier in this book with the metta mediation (see chapter 4) and the 2-10 breathing practice (see chapter 6), we will practice a mindfulness meditation by focusing our awareness on our breath. In our head is the stream of mental activity, wandering in the past and future, thinking all sorts of random things. With mindfulness, the stream of mental phenomena becomes background, and the breath-experience stream becomes foreground. Our awareness is separate and apart from all the rest. Your mind will still be thinking thoughts. Your lungs will still be breathing breaths. But you will bring more awareness to your breath.

## Mindfulness Meditation

1. To begin practice, first sit comfortably with your back straight. It is useful to sit in a chair that helps you keep a straight back, but there is nothing wrong with sitting in a recliner or lying down, though the comfort may lead to more drifting of awareness. If you want to sit cross-legged, rest your bottom on a firm pillow five or six inches thick. This will tilt the pelvis forward, which shifts the body mechanics to a more comfortable posture for an extended period of time. It is not a requirement to sit cross-legged. However, it adds a couple of subtle benefits. First, when you sit with your back straight, you are much more in a state of focused attention. Think of a soldier at attention. Second, we rarely sit this way in modern culture. For this reason, arranging our body in this posture supports the practice. It might sound a little dumb, but when I am sitting cross-legged, palms up with thumbs touching, and back straight, it's like: *Oh yeah, I'm supposed to be meditating.*
2. You also can comfortably lay your hands folded in your lap, thumbs touching, palms up. Placing your hands in the same position each time has another subtle advantage. Over time, you find that simply placing your hands in this position will cue a peaceful response that you often associate with meditating.
3. Breathe in whatever fashion feels comfortable for you.
4. Slowly bring your breath to the foreground of your awareness. Let your thoughts fade into the background. Mentally whisper

"in" on the inhalation and "out" on the exhalation. Try to stretch out the whisper to cover the complete breath cycle: In . . . out . . . Our awareness is now focused on the breath. Breath is what we are experiencing in the present moment. An added benefit is that you get practice in grounding yourself in the here and now, or what is sometimes called the "one-point."

5. Focus on the breath with a certain playful seriousness. You might imagine that you are on a game show. You are in the finals. A million dollars depends on staying focused on the in-out of your breath. At some point in your practice, the game show host will shout: "In or Out!" If you are thinking about what to have for lunch, you just lost a million dollars! The idea is that you are trying to generate a firm intention to follow the in-out of your breath. At the same time, have a gentle playfulness toward the whole thing.

6. You may notice that something in your mind will quickly start tugging at your awareness, trying to pull it into the thought stream. When this happens, you can add in counting your breath cycle: as you inhale and exhale, mentally whisper *In . . . out . . . 1, in . . . out . . . 2, in . . . out . . . 3*, and so on. If you lose track of the count, it will serve as an automatic alert that your awareness has been captured.

7. When your awareness drifts, gently redirect it back to your breath and reset to 1. Don't beat yourself up if you often drift. This is natural at first. If you drift and lose the count and then say to yourself, *I can't do this. It's too hard. I'm the worst meditator ever.* . . . These are just more thoughts. *They are only thoughts.* Part of the practice is realizing that thoughts are merely weird ephemeral things that we don't want to give too much weight to. If you continue to practice, you gradually find that you can go longer and longer without losing the count.

8. Start with five minutes at first. Then try ten to fifteen minutes. Don't be hard on yourself. Be serious but gentle.

Pema Chödrön, an American Tibetan-Buddhist nun who has written many books, stresses approaching meditation with a sense of loving-kindness toward ourselves. Meditation is not intended to get rid of anything. We can still be crazy, angry, or full of feelings of unworthiness. "Meditation practice isn't about trying to throw ourselves away and become something better," she explains. "It's about befriending who we are already. The ground of practice is you or me or whoever we are right now, just as we are. That's what we come to know with tremendous curiosity and interest" (Chödrön, 2002, p.12).

She explains further that curiosity involves being gentle, precise, and open. The practice is approached with a good-heartedness toward ourselves. Precision means seeing clearly, without fearing what's there. Openness means being able to let go. She encourages us to "lighten up" when meditating. Follow the instructions carefully, but be gentle. "Let the whole thing be soft. Breathing out, touch your breath as it goes. Sense the breath going out into a big space and dissolving" (p.19).

## Variations of Basic Practice

Once you get the hang of basic practice, you can make some modifications to deepen your practice, similar to adding more weight to an exercise as your muscles get stronger. Here are modifications that can lead you through deepening and strengthening your meditation practice:

*Try different meditations.* Several excellent resources on the internet provide instructions for basic mindfulness-based meditation practice. There are also good apps for meditation practice. These range from basic timers to guided meditation. Some people prefer a voice to guide them in focusing their awareness. This can aid practice, but try also to practice guiding yourself without an external aid. The skill set that develops from self-guided practice differs from guided meditation.

*Practice without the count.* Maintain the mental whisper, noting the in and out of your breath, but skip counting the cycles. This is a little more challenging, so try this when your attentions is less prone to drifting.

*Practice without the in-out whisper.* This is even more challenging to do. To try this, you should have developed enough focus to be aware when your awareness drifts toward the thought stream.

*Practice staying with the thought stream.* Once you have developed enough control that you are readily aware of when your attention drifts from the breath to the thought stream, you are ready to move your awareness from your breath and intentionally focus on the thought stream. However, try to stay in observer mode. Imagine standing on the shore watching a stream of rushing and tumbling water. On the shore, you are steady and grounded. If you were to fall into the stream and be carried along with the water, it would be a very different experience. Being in observer mode is analogous to standing on the shore and observing the tumbling, rushing stream of your thoughts. To aid you in staying on the shore, try this practice. Rhythmically every four or five seconds notice the thought that is passing by and give that thought a name using the present progressive (i.e., an -*ing* word). For example, I might mentally whisper: *Planning* - - - - - *planning* - - - - - *worrying* - - - - - *remembering* - - - - - *judging* - - - - - *feeling* - - - - - and so on. I might use *thinking* if I cannot find a specific descriptor for the thought.

*Consider your attention capacity.* Some individuals who have compromised attention (such as those who have ADHD or active depression) sometimes have great difficulty sitting in meditation, which then often leads to frustration and giving up on the process. Instead of giving up meditation altogether, try a modification. For example, if you suffer from restlessness and inattention and cannot bear to sit and focus for thirty minutes, try ten or fifteen minutes instead. If that still feels too much, experiment with being intentionally mindful for one or two minutes, but eight to ten times during the day. These brief mindful moments have a cumulative benefit. Use a reminder device to cue you to practice. A random cueing schedule usually works better because we ignore reminders that become too predictable.

### Mindfully "Enlightened"

*Before enlightenment, chopping wood, carrying water. After enlightenment, chopping wood, carrying water.*
*- Zen proverb*

Often our focus is on the ending. We put all of our attention on how things will be when we finally finish. When you achieve your version of "enlightenment," you will still need to do the same things as you continue living.

When we can stay focused in the moment, we no longer feel compelled to watch the clock and look toward the next thing. When you are fully present in whatever your work may be, you may find that your work is no longer a burden. No matter how menial the task may seem, practicing mindfulness and the work at hand will help you develop a habit of always doing your best. Even after you finally achieve "enlightenment," there is still carrying water and chopping wood. The tasks remain the same, but we look at them differently.

# CBT and Right Mindfulness

Our mind can be in different "modes." A common one is analytical mode. This is the mode we usually use to solve problems. It takes the form of *A should be B. How do I close the gap?* A is the current situation, B is the preferred situation, and how can I influence this situation so it moves from A to B? Analytical mode is helpful for solving scientific problems, fixing things, and finishing our work.

Mindful mode is different. It does not take the form of *A should be B*. It is simply A. Not "A should be something else," just A. When in mindful mode, I am fully engaged in the experience of the present moment without judging that moment harshly—I don't put a narrative on top of the experience. Not that I do not judge the present situation at all. But the judgment is a simple noting of whether the moment is pleasant, unpleasant, or neutral. This differs from perceiving the current situation through the lens of an elaborate narrative.

Neither mode is necessarily superior to the other. The usefulness of the mode depends on the context. Analytical mode is helpful for solving problems. However, some problems are not amenable to analytical mode. The more we try to close the gap, the wider it gets. This happens when we overanalyze. The more we try to think our way out of the situation, the more the problem propagates. This is likely a situation that is more amenable to mindfulness.

As we reviewed in the chapter on Right Thought, sometimes we can identify a distorted thought and reframe it into a more useful one. Other times, it is more beneficial to gently hold the immediate experience in our awareness. This is often true for experiences involving our emotions and intimacy. Some feelings need to be gently held and observed without doing anything. Often what is required with intimacy is simple to be fully present.

Mindfulness is a powerful counterweight to anxiety. When we are anxious, our thoughts lean forward into the future. I become obsessed with how the road is going to unfold. *I just know that the meeting will not go well. What if no one shows up for the party? What if I get sick and die? Who will take care of my children?* When we start thoughts with "what if," we are contemplating the future. It is natural to feel compelled to answer questions that we ask ourselves. That is when we fill in the blank of uncertainty that is the future with a story. But the story often generates anxiety. There is an old saying: "If your well-being leaves you, it is hiding from you in the present moment and that is where you should go look for it."

Mindfulness is also a powerful counterweight to depression. When we experience depression, our thoughts are often leaning toward the past. We replay events to which we have attached regret; we revisit losses or traumatic experiences. Mindfulness helps us to transform regrets into intentions. When we realize the past is no longer, we can form intentions that move us forward from the present. By practicing mindfulness, we realize the temporary nature of all things, which helps us to gradually find our peace with loss. When traumatic memories are triggered, mindfulness is how we find our way back to the present.

Mindfulness practices help us develop "observer mode." When we are settled into simple awareness, we are much less likely to have an unnecessary stress response. The 3-column technique (see chapter 4, Right Thought) helps to cultivate observer mode because we first write down our thoughts, and then go back and read what we wrote. When we are reading our recorded thoughts, we are more in observer mode and able to assess our thinking more critically. To develop a calm mind, it is important to be a good observer of what your mind is doing at any given moment.

When we discussed breathing techniques for down-regulating arousal (see 2–10 Breathing in chapter 6, Right Action) the purpose of the technique was to intentionally try to bring about a result. We want to breathe in a certain fashion to create conditions to evoke a relaxation response. However, with mindfulness-based meditation, it is important to approach the practice without trying to "make" something happen, such as relaxing, being peaceful, grabbing enlightenment, or getting your Zen on. Instead of forcing something to happen, have a mindset of just observing what is happening. One helpful mental approach is that when you meditate, you are practicing being a good observer. Sometimes you might observe that during your practice you feel peaceful and centered, other times you are tense with busy thoughts, other times sleepy. Just try to pay close attention to what is going on. Be gentle with yourself without trying to force anything.

## Brain Changes and Mindfulness Practices

In a study looking at brain changes in individuals who meditate, the researchers conducted MRI scans of participants who had completed an eight-week course of mindfulness practice. The results showed significant shrinkage in the amygdala, the brain's "fight or flight" center. This primitive region of the brain initiates the body's response to stress, fear, and emotion. Additionally, they discovered that as the amygdala shrinks, the prefrontal cortex becomes thicker. This area of the brain is associated with higher-order functions such as awareness, concentration, and decision-making.

The MRI scans also showed changes in how often the area of the amygdala and the prefrontal cortex are activated together. This is called *functional connectivity*. In explaining the results, the researchers wrote that mindfulness practice increases one's ability to recruit higher-order, prefrontal cortex regions to downregulate lower-order brain activity. What's more, the connections get stronger as the number of hours of meditation practice increases. Meditation it seems, helps us develop the capacity to use the more thoughtful parts of our brain to override our primitive response to stress (Taren et al., 2013).

If generalized anxiety disorder (GAD) is successfully treated, relevant biomarkers should change, supporting the impact of treatment and suggesting improved resilience to stress. One study looked at adults with GAD who were randomized to receive instruction in either mindfulness-based stress reduction (MBSR) or attention control. MBSR participants had a significantly greater reduction in adrenocorticotropic hormone (ACTH) compared to control participants. Similarly, the MBSR group had a greater reduction in inflammatory cytokine concentrations. This study provided the first combined hormonal and immunological evidence that MBSR may enhance resilience to stress (Hoge et al., 2018).

Brain imaging research has shown that mindfulness practices, such as meditation, can have a positive effect on pain management. Studies using functional magnetic resonance imaging (fMRI) have shown that mindfulness practices can lead to changes in the activity of certain brain regions, such as the anterior cingulate cortex and the insula, that are involved in the processing of pain. Research has also shown that mindfulness practices can lead to changes in how the brain responds to pain, such as increased activity in brain regions associated with regulating emotions and decreased activity in regions associated with the experience of pain. Overall, the research suggests that mindfulness practices may help to reduce the perception of pain and improve the ability to cope with pain.

These brain imaging studies bring together practices that are thousands of years old and determine scientifically exactly why they result in a positive benefit. I remember talking about meditation with a supervisor back in graduate school, asking if he thought it might be beneficial for the patient I was working with who was struggling with stress. His reply was basically: "No, that is mostly just New Age foo-foo stuff." How the times change with science!

## Being Mindful of Duality

We have covered many aspects of being mindful of our thoughts and how they relate to our well-being or lack of well-being. Under some circumstances, we can experience a duality in our mind, when it seems to give us two very different messages at the same time.

One example would be when someone experiences a panic attack. One part of the brain in the neighborhood of the amygdala is giving a signal that the current circumstance is dangerous and activating the fight-or-flight response. Meanwhile, the area of the brain involving the frontal lobes looks around and notices that there is nothing going on. The frontal lobes are the logical, thinking parts of our brains. This duality often causes people to feel as though either the physical sensations must indicate something seriously physically wrong (so let's go to the ER) or they must be going crazy. The duality results from different areas of the brain sending different signals for us to process.

Another example of this phenomenon occurs with obsessive-compulsive disorder. One area of the brain is generating a thought that is experienced as unwanted and ego-dystonic. This thought establishes a circuit linked to the anxiety centers of the brain that fires repetitively. Again, the frontal lobes notice these signals, but consider them irrational. The person experiences that they are being pulled in two different directions. They can't deny the thought and the resulting anxiety, but yet the situation seems completely irrational. Mindfulness can be a strong counterweight in this experience.

When you gently hold the duality in awareness without resisting or acting on the thought, its power diminishes. Clearly label the thought as OCD. Not with a harsh judgement of *Go away! I hate you!* Instead, adopt a stance of loving recognition. *I breathe in, recognizing this thought as OCD. I breathe out knowing all is well.*

Experiencing traumatic stress as a child can also cause this sensation of duality. When a child experiences traumatic stress, such as physical or sexual abuse, the memories of these events get stored differently than routine memories or even negative experiences that are not traumatic. When traumatic memories are activated, the associated emotions can be activated as well. This will often lead to the person re-experiencing the trauma as a flashback.

Other situations can evoke an overall "feeling" that one often experienced as a child. Situations that have enough similarity to events experienced while growing up can put the person back into the place of feeling that they are that child again, sometimes even to the point of physically feeling small. For example, a child might have been often scolded and shamed by her father. Later, now an adult, when publicly scolded by her boss, she might have a physical sensation of feeling unpleasantly like a child again. Or a child who was sexually abused by a caretaker may have developed the response of freezing when touched inappropriately. Later in life, when someone crosses their sexual boundaries they may experience the same freeze response, despite being an assertive, independent, capable adult. Another child might be physically and emotionally abused by a caretaker who cycled between being abusive and overly attentive. As an independent, assertive adult, she may puzzle as to why she stays in a relationship with a toxic boyfriend who exhibits the same dynamics. She feels frustrated, feeling helpless like a child, in stark contrast to how she usually feels.

This duality, where at once the person experiences their world as an adult but also re-experiences very real feelings experienced as a child, is sometimes referred to as the "inner-child," which is a shorthand way of referring to the collections of memories, feelings, and worldview internalized as a child.

For this duality, mindfulness can be a very effective coping mechanism. If I am struggling with the mental problem of aversion, I will fight the feeling of duality. This is like being confronted with the younger version of yourself and saying, *Get away from me, kid. You bother me.* Ignoring, rejecting, shaming are not beneficial ways of interacting with children. Looking at the experience mindfully is more like gently holding hands with your inner child, offering reassurance, saying, *Hello, inner child. How are you today? I know you're anxious or upset, but it's okay. I've got this.*

## The Connection between Gratitude and Well-Being

In chapter 4, Right Thought, we explored a cognitive bias called the negativity bias. Mindfulness is a way of overcoming the negativity bias. If you recall, through evolution we have become hardwired to focus on what's not right, not as it should be, or not as we prefer it to be. This negativity bias offers us an advantage in environments where there are dangerous creatures trying to eat us. However, it is not so useful in our modern environment. The focus on what's not right leaves us preoccupied in a day filled with annoying hassles that stress us out unnecessarily. A counter to this built-in bias is gratitude practice.

Gratitude practice entails being mindful of all the things that you appreciate, are thankful for, are operating normally, and so forth, that often become "background noise" because they are not a problem. Often what is "out of specifications" ("out of spec" for short) is always in the foreground. Things "out of spec" capture our attention. The practice is to allow these things to fade to the background and practice pulling things that are "in spec" into the foreground.

One study examined gratitude and well-being under three experimental conditions. One group was asked to journal about negative events or hassles they experienced each day. A second group was asked to journal about the things for which they were grateful or thankful. The third group logged neutral life events. Participants were required to journal either daily or weekly. Across the various study conditions, the gratitude group consistently showed higher well-being in comparison with the other two study conditions (Emmons & McCullough, 2003).

Another study explored the effect of gratitude on depression and coping efforts in stressed and depressed subjects. Gratitude was found to be a strong protective factor. If we enhance our practice of gratitude, it can help protect us when we are at a low point (Krysinska, 2015). Another study found that even when controlling for personality, a high level of gratitude has a strong positive impact on psychological well-being, self-esteem, and depression (Lin, 2017).

## Gratitude and Loss

Loss seems to be part of life, the dissatisfying part. We want things to be permanent, but they always change. When we experience the loss of something we value, it is natural to experience the suffering of grief.

When we experience grief, the three poisons fill our mind. Desire: *I don't want my loved one to be gone. I want things back the way they were before.* Aversion: *I can't stand the way I feel. This feels bad. I want it to stop.* Ignorance: *Why does my loved one have to die?* When I feel grief, I feel like crying, but there is a lump in my throat. The lump in my throat is my aversion to feeling sad. I don't want to acknowledge feeling sad. *What will make this feeling go away? I want to hold my loved one again.* This is not possible, so I want what is not possible.

As I was writing this book, my beloved dog Bear passed away. He was a King Shepherd that many called the Gentle Giant. He was my best friend. He was only about six years old and in good health. Three weeks before he died, he had what we thought was a simple stomach bug. The vet did some tests and found he had a large tumor on his spleen. The vet estimated he had at the most six months to live. Unfortunately, he had only three weeks. He took his last breath while lying on my lap. I felt the grief of the loss. My heart felt tight. I cried, while also struggling with the lump in my throat. I found it extra hard because our other dogs died when they were at an advanced age and in declining health, allowing us time to prepare for the inevitable loss. Sudden losses are often more difficult because we are suddenly, abruptly reminded that nothing is permanent.

It is normal to feel grief when we experience a loss. But it is important to understand that there is a difference between experiencing grief and *suffering* from experiencing grief. The suffering can be lessened by addressing the three poisons. I can notice that my suffering comes from desire, wanting the emptiness to once again be filled. I suffer from trying to push away the painful feelings, instead of accepting them as part of life when you are lovingly connected to things outside of yourself. I can remind myself of the underlying impermanence of all things and let go of the clinging when something changes.

I can try to do those things, however difficult it is. But I still have a sense of loss and a feeling of emptiness. This empty feeling comes from focusing on what is missing, the absence, the hole in what once was. One thing that can help to fill in the hole is gratitude practice. Gratitude practice entails shifting our focus from what is missing to what is present. When we struggle with loss, what is missing becomes foreground and what is present becomes background. Gratitude reverses this perspective. I am grateful I had a life that included Bear, even if it was only for a few years. I am grateful that he had an illness that did not cause him pain. I am grateful I could hold him while he passed, knowing that he felt love when he took his last breath. I am grateful for all the funny, enjoyable memories of life with the gentle giant. I am grateful that, for now, we still have our other dog Gracie as part of our lives.

## Three Good Things Exercise

Gratitude practice is a simple and effective way to boost your well-being and happiness. This exercise involves reflecting on three good things that happened to you during the day and why they happened. It has been popularized by positive psychology researchers and practitioners, including Dr. Martin Seligman and Dr. Robert Emmons. Here's how you can do it:

1. Take a few minutes at the end of each day to reflect on three good things that happened to you during the day. These can be big or small things, such as having a delicious meal, receiving a compliment, or enjoying a beautiful sunset. You can also pick three things that you were grateful to realize were part of your life that day.
2. Write each of these three things in a journal or notebook. Be as specific as possible about what happened and why you are grateful for it.
3. Take a moment to reflect on why these good things happened. Did you do something to create them, or were they just good luck? Acknowledge any role you played in creating these positive experiences.
4. Finally, take a moment to feel gratitude for these good things. Close your eyes, take a deep breath, and visualize each of the three things in your mind. Allow yourself to feel grateful for each of them and try to savor the positive emotions that come with them.

By practicing gratitude regularly, you can train your brain to focus on the positive aspects of your life and cultivate a more optimistic outlook. Gratitude practice is not about cultivating a pollyannish mindset where everything is puppies and rainbows and you have no problems. It is not about toxic positivity. It is a practice of balancing out our natural tendency to have a negativity bias. Yes, we may have many problems, but there are also puppies and rainbows.

## The Path Forward . . .

Mindfulness is being fully present and aware of what's going on in our immediate experience and in our mind. It is a critical component of the Eightfold Path because if we are not paying attention, we cannot properly practice. We learned it is a skill that can be developed by anyone willing to practice. Mindfulness-based practices have been shown to result in favorable physical changes in the brain. These practices also help us overcome the naturally hardwired tendency toward negativity bias. Now, where do we go from here?

# Part V

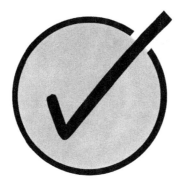

# The Practice

# 11

# CONTINUING ON THE MINDFUL PATH

*An old Cherokee is teaching his grandson about life. "A fight is going on inside me," he tells the boy. "It is a terrible fight, and it is between two wolves.*
*"One is evil—he is anger, envy, sorrow, regret, greed, arrogance, self-pity, guilt, resentment, inferiority, lies, false pride, superiority, and ego."*
*He continued, "The other is good—he is joy, peace, love, hope, serenity, humility, kindness, benevolence, empathy, generosity, truth, compassion, and faith.*
*"The same fight is going on inside you—and inside every other person, too."*
*The grandson thought about it for a minute and then asked his grandfather, "Which wolf will win?"*
*The old Cherokee replied, "The one you feed."*

The story above reflects the reality that, as human beings, we have two sides to our nature and two paths we can follow. We have a nature that can experience both suffering and well-being. We can walk a path that nurtures anger, envy, hate, self-pity, and arrogance. We can also walk a path that nurtures joy, love, humility, kindness, truth, and compassion. Each moment of each day, we face a fork in the road. Which path do you prefer to follow? Which wolf are you going to feed?

We have been exploring the nature of suffering. A good argument can be made that suffering is a part of life. Because we are human, we want things, dislike being uncomfortable, and have trouble seeing things as they are. Added on top of our baseline level of suffering that seems inescapable is an extra layer we cause ourselves. Buddhist practices and CBT seek to identify these sources of suffering and change them in the service of cultivating a more peaceful state for ourselves and those around us.

It seems wise to see reality for how it is, even if seeing it makes us uncomfortable. We seem to be more well when we are aligned with reality instead of twisting it to serve our ego or to fight off uncomfortable feelings. That usually leads to even more suffering. It is wise to understand that a lot of suffering comes from extreme views or behaviors. We do better operating from a centered, middle position. We can adapt to situations more effectively if we recognize things are not permanent. We also become less likely to get out of alignment with reality when we recognize how deceptive our perceptions can be. It is wise to understand how limited we are as human beings in our ability to see things as they are when they are filtered through our perception. We do well when we understand that the ego is an illusion and that seeing ourselves as a separate, permanent self can lead to much suffering. We struggle when we don't realize the difference between what is unbounded and what has limits.

We noted that it is important to align our thoughts with these understandings. When we do that, everything flows easily. We have thoughts of loving-kindness toward ourselves and others, we experience more peace. We explored various ways we can be more mindful of thoughts that generate suffering and how to change them. When we cultivate thoughts in alignment with seeing things as they are, we are cultivating wisdom.

To put this wisdom into practice, we have to apply it in a way that cultivates well-being in ourselves and others. If we have thoughts aligned with how things are, our speech will reflect understanding how things are. With wisdom, our speech will be helpful and kind to others. It will not create ill-will or discord. When our actions are aligned with seeing things as they are, and with healthy thoughts and speech, we will behave with others in a way that is loving and kind. We will treat others ethically. We will engage in actions that reduce suffering in ourselves or others, even if it seems counterintuitive. We will extend our wisdom and ethical mindset toward others when we go out into the world and make a living. How we make a living gives us multiple avenues to engage with others that cultivate well-being in them and ourselves as well.

Keeping track of all of this takes effort. I must make an effort on the journey. The fairies will not deliver well-being to me or those around me. I must cultivate it. It takes work, but the work need not be a burden. Applying wisdom and loving-kindness toward others takes work, but should have a sense of gentleness to it. As I make efforts, I can also explore limits. I have found that healthy stuff tends to be easy. Dysfunctional stuff tends to be complicated and hard. I often tell my patients that I will never invite them to do something harder than what they are already doing. The mindful path is often the easier path.

We also explored mental discipline. It is a challenge to keep the various aspects of the journey in mind. Sometimes I must concentrate and be able to be focused without being distracted. I must understand various ways my concentration can be compromised. I must also have a broad ability to be anchored to the present moment without judgement. We explored various ways of building up this "mental muscle" so it can support the rest of the practice.

Congratulations on your continuing journey of mindful living and well-being. Remember that change is a process, and it takes time and effort to see progress. But with dedication and perseverance, you can achieve your goals.

I encourage you to continue exploring the practices and concepts outlined in this book, and to seek additional resources that resonate with you. There are many excellent books, courses, and teachers available that can help deepen your understanding and support your growth.

Remember to be kind to yourself, and to approach your journey with a sense of curiosity and openness. There will be ups and downs, but every step you take is an opportunity for growth and learning.

Thank you for entrusting me with this part of your journey, and I wish you all the best in your continued path toward greater well-being and happiness. I hope you have found worthwhile my humble effort to explore a pathway to reducing stress, anxiety, depression, and suffering. **_Until next time, have good practice!_**

*We have to let go of the life we planned to accept the one that is waiting for us.*
*–Joseph Campbell*

Thank you for reading my book, I hope you enjoyed it as much as I enjoyed writing it. Won't you please consider leaving a review? Even just a few words would help others decide if the book is right for them.

I've made it super simple: just click this link and you'll travel to the Amazon review page for this book where you can leave your review.

Best regards and thank you in advance:

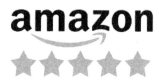

*https://www.amazon.com/dp/B0C3WK6FNJ*

# BIBLIOGRAPHY

Abbasi B, Kimiagar, M, Sadeghniiat, K, Shirazi, M M, Hedayati, M, & Rashidkhani, B. (2012). The effect of magnesium supplementation on primary insomnia in elderly: A double-blind placebo-controlled clinical trial. *Journal of Medical Sciences, Dec. 17*(12), 1161–1169.

Ahn, W. (2022). *Thinking 101: How to Reason Better to Live Better.* Flatiron Books.

Ariely, D. (2008). *Predictably Irrational.* Harper Perenial.

Beck, A. (1967). *Depression: Causes and Treatment.* University of Pennsylvania Press.

Bhagwagar, Z. &. (2020). The neurobiology of serotonergic antidepressants in obsessive-compulsive disorder. *International Journal of Neuropsychopharmacology, 23*(3), 131–143.

Burklund, L J, Creswell, D, Irwin, M R, & Lieberman, M D. (2014, March 24). *The common and distinct neural bases of affect labeling and reappraisal in healthy adults.* Retrieved from Frontiers of Psychology: https://www.ncbi.nlm.nih.gov/pmc/articles/ PMC3970015/

Burns, D. (1980). *Feeling Good: The New Mood Therapy.* New American Library.

Butler, A C & Beck, J S. (2000). Cognitive therapy outcome: A review of meta-analyses. *Journal of the Norwegian Psychological Association, 37.*

Chang, P P, Ford, D E, Meoni, L A, Wang, N-Y, & Klag, M J. (2002). Anger in young men and subsequent premature cardiovascular disease: The precursors study. *Archives of Internal Medicine, 162*(8), 901–906.

Chödrön, P. (2002). *Comfortable with Uncertainty.* Shambhala.

Csikszentmihalyi, M. (1997). *Finding Flow: The Psychology of Engagement in Everyday Life.* Basic Books.

Duhigg, C. (2014). *The Power of Habit: Why We Do What We Do in Life and Business.* Random House.

Ellis, A. (1962). *Reason and Emotion in Psychotherapy.* Stuart.

Emmons, R A & McCullough, M E. (2003). Counted blessings versus burdens: An experimental investigation of gratitude and subjective well-being in daily life. *Journal of Personality and Social Psychology, 84,* 377–389.

Fischhoff, B. S. (1980). Knowing what you want: Measuring labile values. In Wallsten, T S (Ed.), *Cognitive processes in choice and decision behavior pp. 117-141.* Lawrence Erlbaum.

Fisher, R & Ury, W. (2006). *Getting to Yes (2nd ed.).* Penguin Putnam.

Fjorback, L. O. (n.d.). Mindfulness-based intervention in schizophrenia: a randomized controlled trial. *Acta psychiatrica Scandinavica, 124(2), 102-109., 124*(2), 102-109.

Garcia, H. (2017). *Ikigai: The Japanese Secret to a Long and Happy Life.* Penguin Books.

Gethin, R. T. (1998). *The Foundations of Buddhism.* Oxford University Press.

Goldstein, J. (2008). *Cause and Effect: Reflections on The Laws of Karma.* Retrieved from Tricycle: The Buddhist Review: https://tricycle.org/magazine/cause-and-effect/

Gollwitzer, A. O. (2022). Discordant knowing: A social cognitive structure underlying fanaticism. *Journal of Experimental Psychology: General, 151*(11), 2846–2878.

Goodman, W. (2022). *Toxic Positivity: Keeping It Real in a World Obsessed with Being Happy.* Penguin Randomhouse.

Gottman, J, & Gottman, J. (2008). Gottman method of couple therapy. In A. Gurman (Ed.), *Clinical Handbook of Couple Therapy* (pp. 138–164). The Guildfod Press.

Gottman, J. (2000). *The Seven Principles for Making Marriage Work*. Orion.

Greenberger, B & Padesky, C A. (1995). *Mind Over Mood*. Guilford Press.

Gunaratana, B. (2001). *Eight Mindful Steps to Happiness: Walking the Buddha's Path*. Wisdom Publications.

Hanh, T. N. (1998). *The Heart of the Buddha's Thinking*. Parallax Press.

Hanson, R. (2009). *Buddha's Brain: The Practical Neuroscience of Happiness, Love, and Wisdom*. New Harbinger Publications.

Hanstede, M. G. (2008). The effects of a mindfulness intervention on obsessive-compulsive symptoms in a non-clinical student population. *Journal of Nervous Mental Disorders, 196*(10), 776–779.

Hertenstein, E. R. (2012). Mindfulness-based cognitive therapy in obsessive-compulsive disorder: A qualitative study on patients' experiences. *BMC Psychiatry, 12*(185).

Holmes, D. (2017, April 7). *Concerning Right Action and Right Livelihood*. Retrieved from Buddhist Door Global: https://www.buddhistdoor.net/features/concerning-right-action-and-right-livelihood/

Jerath, R, Crawford, M W, Barnes, V A, & Harden, K. (2015). Self-regulation of breathing as a primary treatment for anxiety. *Applied Psychophysiolology: Biofeedback, 40*, 107–115.

Kahneman, D. (2011). *Thinking, Fast and Slow*. Farrar, Straus, and Giroux.

Kanheman, D & Deaton, A. (2010, September). High income improves evaluation of life but not emotional well-being. *Proceeding of the National Academy of Sciences, 107*(38), 1648--16493.

Keown, D. O. (2004). *Buddhism: A Very Short Introduction*. Oxford University Press.

Khong, B. S. (2003). The Buddha teaches an attitude, not an affili ation. In S. R. Segall (Ed.), *Encountering Buddhism: Western Psychology and Buddhist Teachings.* State Unversity of New York Press.

Kozyreva, A, Wineburg, S, Hertwig, R, & Lewandowsky, S. (2022). Critical Ignoring as a Core Competence for Digital Citizens. Retrieved from Current Directions in Psychological Science: https://doi.org/10.1177/09637214221121570

Kross, E V, et al. (2013). Facebook use predicts declines in subjective well-being in young adults. *Plos one, 8(8), e69841.*, 8(8), e69841.

Krysinska, K. L. (2015). Trait gratitude and suicidal ideation and behavior: An exploratory study. *Crisis: The Journal of Crisis Intervention and Suicide Prevention, 36*, 291–296.

Ledi, S. (1977). *The Noble Eightfold Path and Its Factors Explained.* Buddhist Publication Society.

Leventhal, A. W. (2020). Association between social media use and depression among US adolescents. *JAMA, 77*(2), 168-175.

Lewinsohn, P M & Atwood, G E. (1969). Depression: A clinical-research approach. *Psychotherapy: Theory, Research & Practice, 6*(3), 166–171.

Light, N. F. (2022). Knowledge overconfidence is associated with anti-consensus views on controversial scientific issues. *Science Advances, 8*(29).

Lin, C. (2017). The effect of higher-order gratitude on mental well-being: Beyond personality and unifactoral gratitude. *Current Psychology, 36*, 127–135.

Madore K P & Wagner, A D. (2019). Multicosts of Multitasking. *Cerebrum.*

McNeil, B. P. (1982). On the elicitation of prefeences for alternative therapies. *New England Journal of Medicine, 306*, 1259–1262.

Mehta, R. A. (2016). The effects of multitasking on emotional well-being. Social cognitive and affective neuroscience, 11(1), 30-41. *Social cognitive and affective neuroscience, 11*(1), 30-41.

Mlodinow, L. (2009). *The Drunkard's Walk: How Randomness Rules Our Lives.* Vintage.

Nickerson, R. (1998). Confirmation bias: A ubiquitous phenomenon in many guises. *Review of General Psychology, 2*(2), 175–220.

Oremus W, Alcantara, C, Merrill, J B & Galocha, A. (2021, October 26). *How Facebook shapes your feed.* Retrieved from The Washington Post: https://www.washingtonpost.com/technology/interactive/2021/how-facebook-algorithm-works/

Perlis, R H, et al. (2021). Association between social media use and self-reported symptoms of depression in US Adults. *JAMA Network Open, 4*(11).

Rahula, W. (1978). *What the Buddha Taught.* The Gordon Fraser Gallery.

Schmidt, A. (2017, March 6). *PNAS.* Retrieved from https://doi.org/10.1073/pnas.1617052114

Sharif, M. M. (2021). Having too little or too much time is linked to lower subjective well-being. *Journal of Personality and Social Psychology: Personality Processes and Individual Differences*, 1–15.

Siegman, A. (1993). Cardiovascular consequences of expressing, experiencing, and repressing anger. *Journal of Behavioral Medicine, 16*, 539–569.

Soroka, S. F. (2019). Cross-national evidence of a negativity bias in psychophysiological reactions to news. *Proceedings of the National Academy of Sciences, 116*, 18888–18892.

Stancák, A, Pfeffer, D, Hrudová, L, Sovka, P, & Dostálek, C. (1993). Electroencephalographic correlates of paced breathing. *Neuroreport, 4*, 723–726.

Sterner, T. (2012). *The Practicing Mind.* New World Library.

Taren, A A, Creswell, J D, & Gianaros, P J. (2013, May). Dispositional mindfulness co-varies with smaller amygdala and caudate volumes in community adults. *PLOS One, 8*(5).

Tawwab, N. G. (2021). *Set Boundaries, Find Peace: A Guide to Reclaiming Yourself.* TarcherPerigee.

Tversky, A & Kahneman, D. (1973). Availability: A heuristic for judging frequency and probability. *Cognitive Psychology, 5*(2), 207–232.

Twenge, J M, Joiner, T E , Rogers, M L, & Martin, G N. (2018). Increases in depression, suicide-related outcomes, and suicide rates among U.S. adolescents after 2010 and links to increased new media screen time. *Clinical Psychological.*

Vaillant, G. E. (2012). *Triumphs of experience: The men of the Harvard Grant Study.* Harvard University Press.

Vaish, A. G. (2008). Not all emotions are created equal: The negativity bias in social-emotional development. *Psychological Bulletin, 134*(3), 383–403.

Vaughn, S. (2021, October 5). History of DBT: Origins and foundations. Retrieved from Psychotherapy Academy: https://psychotherapyacademy.org/dbt/history-of-dialectical-behavioral-therapy-a-very-brief-introduction/

Verrier, R L & Mittleman, M A. (1996). Life-threatening cardiovascular consequences of anger in patients with coronary heart disease. *Cardiology Clinics, 14*(2), 289–307.

Wahl, K. (2013). Managing obsessive thoughts during brief exposure: An experimental study comparing mindfulness-based strategies and distraction in obsessive-compulsive disorder. *Cognitive Therapy & Research, 37*(4), 752–761.

Willing, A E, et al. (2019). Brazilian Jiu Jitsu Training for US Service Members and Veterans with Symptoms of PTSD . *Military Medicine, 184*(11-12).

Zaccaro A, Piarulli, A, Laurino, M, Garbella, E, Menicucci, D, Neri, B, & Gemignani, A. (2017, September 7). *How breath-control can change your life: A systematic review on psycho-physiological correlates of slow breathing.* Retrieved from Frontiers: https://www.frontiersin.org/journals/human-neuroscience

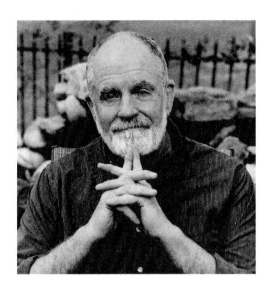

# ABOUT THE AUTHOR

Dr. Jones is a clinical psychologist practicing in Houston for over thirty-five years. He has maintained a private practice with his wife, Lesli, also a clinical psychologist. Understanding that therapy is very personal and everyone's journey is different, Dr. Jones takes an eclectic approach to treatment. His lifelong interest in Buddhist philosophy contributed to his interest in clinical psychology.

He has studied several martial arts most of his life. He is a Brazilian Jiujitsu black belt and continues to train regularly. Dr. Jones has completed many marathons as well as 100-mile ultramarathons. He enjoys applying lessons learned from these pursuits as well as from his many patients over the years to his practice of psychotherapy.

Dr. Jones is a husband of thirty-five years, a proud father to three adult children, and a grandfather. He lives with his wife, Lesli, and their German Shepherd rescue dog, Gracie.

Printed in Great Britain
by Amazon

32970460R00116